Aromatherapy in Essence

by

Chrissie Wildwood
LLSA (hons) MCH

Published by

Masada Ltd
Aldborough. York,
North Yorkshire. YO51 9ES
http://www.books.masada.ltd.uk

ISBN 0-9538574-0-9

Cover design by M A Newbould
Harrogate Photographic Laboratories
Telephone 01423 501066
www.photo-labs.com

Printed in Great Britain by
York Publishing Services Ltd
York YO31 7ZQ
Telephone 01904 431 213 Fax 01904 430 868
www.yps-publishing.co.uk

Contents

Essential Oil Profiles explored within this publication

L

M

N

O

P

R

S

T

V

Y

About the author

Chrissie Wildwood LLSA (hons) MCH[1]

Chrissie Wildwood qualified in aromatherapy and massage in 1983, having studied at The London School of Aromatherapy. In 1986 she became vice-principal of the school, but resigned after a year in order to develop her aromatherapy practice in Wales and to concentrate on her writing career. She went on to train in counselling, subtle healing techniques, flower remedies, meditation and deep relaxation therapy with the College of Healing in Malvern, gaining a diploma from the college in 1987. Solely for research purposes she has also trained in hypnotherapy (1998).

Chrissie is a freelance internationally known health and specialist writer / lecturer[2] on the subject of aromatherapy. She has also taken part in numerous television and radio shows. As well as being a consultant for several companies producing natural health care products, she is the author of 12 books[3] on aromatherapy, flower remedies and related subjects, including the best-selling Bloomsbury Encyclopaedia of Aromatherapy. She is also a member of NORA (Natural Oils Research Association).

Above all Chrissie is recognised as one who adopts and imparts a practical, common sense approach to Aromatherapy and its broader associated subjects.

[1] LLSA (hons)   THE LONDON SCHOOL OF AROMATHERAPY
     MCH   THE COLLEGE OF HEALING
[2] UK, USA, Canada and Japan
[6] Translated into over 10 different languages

Acknowledgement

Thank you Jon for all your hard work in setting all the text and compiling the indexes, and for painstakingly seeing this book through the many stages prior to publication. Above all, thank you for coming up with the idea in the first place!

Chrissie

Chrissie Wildwood

Editor's Comment

The development of blending skills often overlooked. Certainly in my years as a supplier of aromatherapy products it was always evident that most potential sources of learning and advancement failed to explore and develop this important and most rewarding aspect of aromatherapy. Indeed I would say that it was perhaps one of the most frequently discussed topics, among therapist, students and home users alike. They simply wanted to learn more, and the information available was just not offering enough.

Aromatherapy in Essence has been allowed to develop quite naturally. From the initial concept of a simple, quick, common sense reference guide it has blossomed into a comprehensive manual, while still remaining concise and accessible to the general reader.

Chrissie has included comprehensive "Considerations" subsections for the oils which is further supported throughout the first 4 chapters with other vital information for your guidance. With Chrissie's help it is now possible for you experience an enhanced enjoyment and gain greater personal benefit from your use of essential oils.

Aromatherapy in Essence is therefore of great value to professional, student and home user alike.

Jon Beavis-Harrison

Editor

Note to the reader

Neither the author nor publisher may be held responsible for misadventure resulting from the misuse of essential oils, or any other therapeutic method mentioned in this publication. While the author has endeavoured to ensure that the contents of this book are accurate, it can not be read or regarded as a substitute for professional medical advice.

Where there is doubt about how to use an essential oil, or if there is concern regarding the suitability of home treatment for a particular ailment, seek the advice of a qualified aromatherapist.

Should symptoms persist despite sensible use of essential oils, it is important to seek medical advice and to mention that aromatherapy has been used. It may also be necessary to provide information on the precise aromatherapeutic preparation(s) employed. Therefore it is advisable and good practice to keep accurate records of oils used, noting any positive or negative effects resulting.

NB.

NB. Reference should also be made to Homoeopathic considerations under Essential Oil Safety Precautions - page 18.

CHAPTER 1

THE ROOTS OF AROMATHERAPY

Aromatherapy is the therapeutic use of essential oils extracted from certain aromatic plants and trees. Treatment involves applying these oils to the body - or simply inhaling them - to improve health and promote an inner sense of well-being.

Since the beginning of history, aromatic plants have played an important role in traditional medicine throughout the world. But it was the French cosmetic scientist Rene-Maurice Gattefossé who coined the term 'Aromatherapy', which was the title of his first book on the subject published in 1937. He was particularly intrigued by the remarkable antibiotic and antiseptic properties of essential oils.

Other aromatherapy pioneers followed Gattefossé's lead, the most notable being Dr Jean Valnet, a French army surgeon who advocated essential oils in the treatment of soldiers wounded in battle. Later he used the oils, in conjunction with herbal medicine, to treat patients in psychiatric hospitals. Many of these people were eventually weaned off powerful drugs, the side-effects of which had been found to complicate their distressing conditions. Valnet describes such treatments in his book, The Practice of Aromatherapy, a translation from the French which was first published in 1982 and has since become a classic in its field.

It was the Austrian-born cosmetologist Marguerite Maury who developed the art of aromatherapy massage, based on the techniques employed by traditional healers in Tibet. In the early 1960s she introduced aromatherapy clinics to Britain. Although her treatments were geared to beauty therapy she knew that aromatherapy went much deeper. Her clients reported pleasant side-effects such as deeper sleep, an improved mental state and increased vitality. Most aromatherapists outside France continue to follow Maury's lead and incorporate massage therapy as the mainstay of treatment with essential oils.

French aromatherapy doctors, on the other hand, advocate conventional methods of treatment, which includes prescribing oral doses of encapsulated essential oils, administering them in the form of suppositories and applying them as antiseptic and antifungal agents. In other words, essential oils are treated in much the same way as pharmaceutical drugs. Essential oils, however, are regarded as superior in many ways; not only because they work, but because when skilfully prescribed they are infinitely less toxic than conventional drugs (see Essential Oil Chemistry, page 2).

In recent years aromatherapy (in its many facets) is a recognised and important part of complementary health care, especially in Britain. It's also gaining recognition and a degree of medical acceptance in the USA, Canada, Australia and Japan. Essential oils (the subject of ongoing scientific research) are commonly incorporated as part of an holistic healing plan, supporting the benefits of good nutrition, moderate exercise, relaxation techniques and other important adjuncts to promoting health and vitality. In this context, aromatherapy is successful in relieving a whole host of health problems - from stress to PMS, from respiratory ailments to digestive complaints, and from skin problems to muscular pain. Aromatherapy is beneficial in more serious conditions, but the home-user of essential oils should always seek the advice of a professional aromatherapist - and the co-operation of a medical doctor - before attempting treatment of chronic health problems.

There are many ways to use essential oils. Most aromatherapists favour diluting them in a vegetable carrier oil (such as sweet almond) and applying to the body using skilled but nurturing massage. A wonderful treatment which combines the physical and psychological benefits of massage with the medicinal and mood-enhancing properties of the oils. Add gentle music and a pleasing decor (as many aromatherapists do) and we are nurtured on every level of our being. But what exactly are essential oils, and how do they exert their beneficial effects?

THE NATURE OF ESSENTIAL OILS

Essential oils (also commonly known as essences, aromatic oils or volatile oils) are extracted from various parts of a wide range of aromatic plants and trees. For example, they may be found in the leaves (eucalyptus), roots of grass (palmarosa), flowers (rose), rhizomes or roots (ginger), heartwood (sandalwood), rind (lemon). Not all plants secrete essential oils, which means that scent is not vital to the life of plants in general. When plants do produce an essential oil, there are three main reasons for its presence: to attract pollinating insects; to protect the plant from certain diseases; and to form a vapour veil around the plant during hot weather to protect it from excessive water loss.

Even though they are technically classified as oils, plant essences are quite different from 'fixed' or fatty oils such as sunflower seed or olive. They are highly volatile and will evaporate when left in the open air, and most will not leave a permanent stain on paper. Many have the consistency of water or alcohol - lavender, peppermint and rosemary, for example. Others like sandalwood and vetiver are quite viscous, whereas rose otto is semi solid at room temperature, but becomes liquid with the slightest warmth.

ESSENTIAL OIL CHEMISTRY

The chemistry of essential oils is elaborate. An individual oil may have hundreds of identifiable chemicals, the principle components being a group of complex substances known as terpenes and their compounds or derivatives. This explains why a single essential oil has a wide range of therapeutic actions. However, it's important to remember that essential oils are not simply concentrated versions of herbal medicines (as is commonly believed), for in fact they lack water soluble constituents such as tannins and pectins which are found in the raw plant material.

Nevertheless, the multifarious therapeutic properties of essential oils (and indeed, all plant medicines) results from synergism - an interaction of all its chemical constituents working harmoniously together, so that the effect of the whole becomes greater than the sum of its parts. But drug manufacturers prefer to isolate the 'active principles' of raw plant material and essential oils. This might lead to attempts to synthesise them, or to experiment with changing them slightly to achieve certain desired effects such as increased activity and greater stability. (Incidentally, since chemical drugs can be patented, resulting in higher profits for the manufacturer, there is little incentive to promote essential oils and herbal medicines.) However, the compounds and substances which the drug manufacturers seek to eliminate work in concert with the 'actives', making them more easily utilised by the body. They also buffer the action of what are otherwise powerful chemicals, thus protecting the body from dangerous side-effects.

Moreover, as every chemist knows, it's impossible to replicate a natural chemical. A synthesised drug always carries with it a small percentage of undesirable substances which are not found in nature. What effect some of these new synthetic drugs will have on people in the long term is little understood. But despite the pitfalls of conventional drug therapy, it's important to adopt a balanced viewpoint. Not all essential oils and herbs are without dangerous side-effects. Tansy essential oil, for example, and the herbal remedy foxglove are both potentially lethal unless administered with utmost skill by an aromatherapy doctor or medical herbalist. Moreover, potentially dangerous chemical drugs do have a role to play in health care; for example, in cases of chronic pain and congenital organ dysfunction where conventional treatment may be vital.

PRINCIPAL EXTRACTION METHODS

Steam Distillation

Most essential oils are extracted by steam distillation a process whose basic principles have remained unchanged for centuries - albeit that modern stainless steel distillation equipment is much more efficient. Plant material is placed in the still, and steam is passed through it. The heat and pressure release the essential oil droplets, which then rise with the steam. The aromatic vapour is carried along a closed outlet and is cooled and condensed (turned back to liquid) by being passed through a cold water jacket. The resulting aromatic water is collected in a Florentine flask. The essential oil, being lighter than water, floats on the surface and is later separated. The leftover water (technically known as a hydrolat or hydrosol) remains quite aromatic and can often be used as a therapeutic/cosmetic by-product. Rosewater and orange flower water are two well-known examples.

Expression

A process used to extract the essential oil found in the rind of citrus fruits. Although this was once carried out by hand (by squeezing the rind and collecting the oil in a sponge), machines using centrifugal force are now used instead. However, lime essential oil is more often captured by steam distillation because the expressed version can be highly irritant to skin.

Super Critical Carbon Dioxide (CO_2) Extraction

A process whereby carbon dioxide gas at very high pressure is use to dissolve essential oil from a wide range of plant material. The equipment is massive and extremely expensive, but there are several process plants around the world producing essential oils with an excellent quality of aroma. However, the chemistry of a CO_2 extract is somewhat different from that of a steam distilled oil, and thus should be regarded with a degree of caution. Ginger CO_2, for example, is more likely to irritate sensitive skin. CO_2 aromatics are also considerably more expensive than steam distilled essential oils.

3

Volatile Solvent Extraction

The essential oils of certain flowers such as jasmine, carnation and narcissus, are damaged by the intense heat of steam distillation. To capture such precious fragrances, the plant material undergoes a complicated process involving the use of volatile petro-chemical solvents such as hexane and petroleum ether. The resulting viscous extract is known as an 'absolute'. Absolutes have an excellent quality of aroma, and are thus valued for their mood-enhancing potential. However, they are considerably more expensive than most essential oils.

HOW DO ESSENTIAL OILS WORK?

Research into essential oils reveals that these complex substances are endowed with numerous therapeutic properties (see Aromatic Portraits). Generally speaking, most essential oils are antiseptic; some are antifungal; and a few may be antiviral. When applied externally, there are two main routes by which they may reach the bloodstream. By skin absorption and by inhalation. Whether absorbed through the skin or inhaled, once in the bloodstream essential oils are believed to interact with the body chemistry and exert a pharmacological effect - even though the amount absorbed is very small indeed. According to Gattefossé, essential oils diluted to a degree at which they no longer have an effect on living cultures in the laboratory still have a clear, rapid and beneficial action in the body. Such findings have since been borne out by other researchers investigating the therapeutic properties of essential oils.

Valnet and others have also discovered that blends of certain essential oils are not only more powerful than when used singly, but that the mysterious factor of synergy is at work (as described under Essential Oil Chemistry on page 2). When certain essential oils are blended together they have a mutually enhancing effect on one another, so that the effect of the whole is greater than the sum of its individual parts. This is particularly noticeable with the bactericidal action of essential oils. A blend of clove, thyme, lavender and peppermint, for example, is far more powerful than the biochemist might expect of the blend (taking into account the combined chemical constituents of the oils). Curiously, by mixing more than five essential oils, the effect is sometimes counter-productive. The bactericidal action is weakened.

Quite apart from their pharmacological activity, studies have shown that odour can have a profound effect on our emotions. This is because the olfactory nerves in the upper part of the nose pass directly to the limbic system or 'smell brain'. Although this area of the brain is still largely uncharted territory, we do know that is concerned with our instincts: emotion, intuition, memory, creativity, hunger, thirst, sleep patterns, libido and probably much else besides. Scent, as a result, can evoke memories, feelings and images, or even move us to actions without our even knowing it.

ESSENTIAL OIL QUALITY

Essential oils can vary enormously in price and quality, depending on two main factors: the amount of oil found in the plant material and the integrity of the distillation process. The more oil glands present in the plant, the cheaper the oil, and vice versa. 100 kilos of lavender, for instance, yields almost 3 litres of essential oil; whereas 100 kilos of rose petals surrenders merely half a litre. A poorly distilled oil may smell 'burnt' or 'stewed' as a result of human error (some plants require a shorter distillation process than others). Poorly distilled oils are unreliable as therapeutic products, for their chemistry is somewhat different from usual.

The quality of aroma is also influenced by the vagaries of the climate, geographical location, soil condition, altitude, air quality - and probably many other subtle and interrelated factors as yet unrecognised by science. So the aroma of a genuine essential oil will vary from one harvest to the next, just like the bouquet of a good wine. This also explains why the same named oil is likely to smell somewhat different from one supplier to the next.

The unpredictable variation of aroma, combined with other possible risks such as poor harvests, political conflicts and transportation difficulties, means that the perfume and flavours industries (the main buyers of essential oils) prefer to rely on standardised oils - aromatics which have been altered in the laboratory to meet a required chemical formulation. Such products are categorised as 'commercial' or 'industrial' grade oils. Others may be partially synthetic and labelled 'nature identical'.

Unfortunately, the demand for essential oils (especially lavender, rose, geranium and sandalwood) often exceeds the world supply. Therefore, commercial grade essential oils may well be seeping into the aromatherapy market. Although such oils usually retain a degree of therapeutic activity, as can be demonstrated in the laboratory, this is beside the point. Apart from increased risk of skin reactions and respiratory irritation, the use of 'nature identical', or otherwise adulterated oils, runs counter to the philosophy of aromatherapy. So it's vital to purchase your oils from a reputable supplier (see Suppliers page 125).

WHERE TO BUY ESSENTIAL OILS

Aromatherapists usually purchase essential oils from specialist mail order suppliers, and most firms respond quickly. Since many are also happy to sell small quantities to unqualified essential oil enthusiasts, it's always worth asking an aromatherapist in your area to recommend a supplier. You could also try telephoning an aromatherapy training school to find out which oils they recommend: they may even distribute their own. Good quality oils are also available from certain health food shops, pharmacies and shops specialising in herbs and other natural remedies - but again, it's worth seeking the recommendation of a local aromatherapist.

ALWAYS READ THE LABEL

Top quality essential oils should be labelled 'pure and natural', which means they are unblended and contain no synthetic substances. Since the common names for plants and their essential oils vary from one country to another, the botanical name should always be included on the label. For example, not just 'Lavender', but also Lavandula angustifolia.

Synthetic concoctions aside, there are other oils which are commonly mistaken for top grade products - oils which are labelled 'natural'. Although these oils should be free of synthetic additives, it is legally permissible for such products to be extended with other natural materials. For example, geranium may be stretched with the less expensive palmarosa, and Melissa (a very costly oil) with the isolated component citral, which commonly derives from citronella.

You may also come across a bottle labelled 'Aromatherapy Oil', which usually means it's a mixture of about 2-3 per cent essential oil in a carrier such as grapeseed or almond oil, often with the addition of vitamin E as a preservative. These are fine as ready-mixed massage oils, although an expensive way to enjoy aromatherapy. For instance, a 10 ml bottle (the average size) of a diluted essential oil is barely enough for two face and neck massages, whereas 10 ml of pure essential oil, once correctly diluted, is enough for countless full-body massages.

Another drawback, ready-mixed oils are not concentrated enough to be used by the drop to perfume the bath water - nor indeed, to use in a vaporiser for fragrancing a room. True, one or two oils like rose otto and neroli are very expensive and buying the ready-diluted versions can indeed be a good way to begin experimenting with them. But remember, a little bottle of pure oil goes a very long way, so it's always worth the investment!

COMPARE PRICES

Genuine essential oils are not cheap. Be cautious of ranges where expensive oils such as neroli, rose otto and clary sage are priced at the same rate as relatively inexpensive oils such as lemon or eucalyptus globulus. If in serious doubt about the quality of an essential oil labelled 'pure and natural' contact the Essential Oil Trade Association (EOTA) who may agree to carry out a laboratory test to establish the quality of the oil in question.

CARING FOR YOUR OILS

Essential oils evaporate readily and are easily damaged by light, extremes of temperature and exposure to oxygen in the air. For this reason they are sold in well-stoppered, dark glass bottles. The bottle should be equipped with an accurate integral dropper cap. A poorly designed integral dropper causes the oil to pour out, thus making it impossible to measure the oils accurately.

In ideal conditions most essential oils will keep for several years, although the average shelf life is about two years. However, with the exception of bergamot, expressed (cold-pressed) citrus oils deteriorate within 6-12 months. But all essential oils are vulnerable. The more often you open the bottle, the greater the chance of oxidation - a process whereby a substance is chemically combined with oxygen and its original structure altered or destroyed - as reflected in the deterioration of aroma and possibly a cloudy appearance. As well as the problem of decreased potency, an oxidised (rancid) oil is highly likely to cause skin irritation.
To prolong the life of your oils, store them in a cool, dry, dark place. Essential oils can also be stored in the fridge (enclosed in an airtight food container), although not in the freezer compartment. Citrus oils will turn cloudy if stored in cold conditions, but regain their clarity at room temperature.

STORING MASSAGE OILS, LOTIONS AND POTIONS

Although pure essential oils have a long shelf life, once diluted in a carrier oil, unperfumed cream/lotion or distilled water, their potency begins to diminish after about six weeks, or even sooner unless stored in the fridge. If diluted in a cold-pressed or unrefined vegetable oil, the risk of oxidation is greatly increased. As with pure essential oils, it all depends on how often you open the bottle (or jar). Always keep cold-pressed oils in the fridge, and use up by the best-before date.

Shop-bought aromatherapy massage oils are usually preserved with vitamin E, an antioxidant which helps guard against rancidity. So you might wish to add the contents of 2 vitamin E capsules to every 30 ml of aromatherapy massage oil (pierce the capsules with a pin and squeeze the contents into the aromatherapy blend). If stored in the fridge, this is thought to extend the shelf life to about four months. Contrary to the advice given in most aromatherapy books, it's not advisable to add wheatgerm oil to massage blends in the hope that it will extend the shelf-life of the product (reasons are given below)

Apart from the risk of oxidation, essential oils evaporate when exposed to air. So the Odour Intensity of most bottled aromatherapy blends will quickly diminish. Rather than trying to prolong the life of your blends, however, it's far better to mix just enough oil for each treatment - or perhaps enough to last for up to a week.

THE TRUTH ABOUT WHEATGERM OIL

Most aromatherapy books suggest that to prolong the shelf-life of your massage blends, add up to 15 per cent of wheatgerm oil. The reasoning behind this statement is that wheatgerm oil is high in vitamin E, a natural antioxidant. So by adding it to other vegetable oils, it guards against rancidity. Now, anyone who is familiar with wheatgerm oil, whether it's extracted by volatile solvents or warm compressed, will know that the substance is highly unstable. Therefore it must be kept in the fridge and used up within a few months of opening the bottle. It also smells unpleasant and diminishes the aesthetic value of aromatherapy blends. Quite apart from its smell - and indeed, it's slimy texture - how can something as unstable as wheatgerm oil possibly act as a preservative? It's more likely to have the opposite effect!
In fact, one of the most stable of unrefined vegetable oils is extra virgin olive - an oil which has been used since antiquity. According to a food scientist of my acquaintance, Dr Jennes Kristott of Pura Food Produce Ltd (UK), it is the only unrefined vegetable oil that does not need to be stored in the fridge. And yet, if you check the nutritional charts found in any good text book on nutrition and food values, you will discover that wheatgerm oil contains 30 times more vitamin E than olive oil! Clearly, vitamin E is not the wonder preservative many would have us believe - at least not when found in natural synergy with all the other elements which comprise wheatgerm oil. On the other hand, synthetic vitamin E, such as d-alpha-tocopheryl acetate, is indeed a powerful antioxidant, which is why it is commonly used as an active ingredient and preservative in cosmetics and nutritional supplements.

CHAPTER 2:

DIFFERENT WAYS TO USE ESSENTIAL OILS

Essential oils can be used in a variety of ways to promote health and vitality. They can be used in skin-care preparations, made into massage oils, added to the bath, used in steam inhalations for colds and 'flu, blended into mood-enhancing perfumes and in other ways to enhance our daily lives. To help you choose the right essential oils for healing purposes, refer to the information given in Chapter 4, relevant sections in Chapter 5 Essential Oil Profiles pages 35-115 and the Quick Guide to Essential Oils for Common Ailments on page 116.

AROMATHERAPY MASSAGE

As mentioned earlier, massage is the mainstay of most professional aromatherapy treatments. There is no denying that it can be a truly divine experience, and giving massage can be enjoyable too. Unfortunately, it is beyond the scope of this book to include illustrated massage sequences. In any case, it's impossible to learn massage solely from a book. At some point, you will need to attend classes. You may even decide to embark on an extended study course (see Useful Addresses at the end of this book).

You can of course, massage the oils into your own body and derive benefit from them - especially if applied immediately after a bath or shower, as warmth and moisture facilitate skin absorption. Massage upwards over your whole body (or as much of it as you can reach), always towards the heart to improve the circulation. Generally, brisk hand-over-hand movements are enlivening, while long, slow strokes are relaxing.

MIXING MASSAGE OILS

Essential oils intended for massage need to be diluted in a vegetable carrier/base oil such as sweet almond or sunflower (see Quick Guide to Carrier Oils, page 11). A cold-pressed vegetable oil will have a higher vitamin content. However, such oils are not always suitable for sensitive skin which may react to the various additional elements found in unrefined oils. If in doubt, carry out a 24-hour patch test (see page 19).

Although standard dilutions are given in the chart below, it is important to remember that certain essential oils are more odoriferous than average, and thus smaller quantities are normally used to achieve the desired result (i.e. 0.5 to 1 per cent). If you cannot judge the Odour Intensity of a particular oil (by using your nose), refer to the specific blending advice included in the Essential Oil Profiles – chapter 5.

EASY MEASURES FOR MASSAGE OILS:

Mixing enough oil for a single treatment

Mix the oils in a saucer or little dish. Use a 5ml plastic medicine spoon (available from pharmacies) to measure the base oil, as ordinary teaspoons generally hold less than 5 ml. For a full body massage, you will need about 4-6 teaspoons of oil (a little more if the skin is hairy or very dry).

For a facial massage, you will need as little as 1 teaspoon of oil. Since the skin of the face is usually more sensitive than the rest of the body, it is important to make up a separate facial oil using less essential oil (see Dilution Guide below).

Mixing larger quantities of massage oil

For larger quantities of massage oil, inexpensive dark glass bottles suitable for storing massage blends are obtainable from pharmacies. The capacity in mls is usually imprinted into the glass on the base of the bottle. The 50 ml and 100 ml sizes are the most useful. When filling the bottles with base oil, a small kitchen funnel will ease the process. Funnel half the required amount of base oil into the bottle, add the essential oils and shake well to disperse, then fill the bottle almost to the top with base oil and shake again.

Dilution Guide

Low dilution for facial massage and for use during pregnancy

Mix the essential oils to a 1 per cent dilution:
1 drop essential oil per teaspoon (5ml) carrier oil

Normal dilution for body massage

Mix the essential oils to a 2 or 3 per cent dilution:
2 per cent dilution = 2 drops essential oil per teaspoon (5 ml) carrier oil
3 per cent dilution = 3 drops essential oil per teaspoon (5ml) carrier oil

Extremely low dilution for very sensitive skin and babies.

N.B. But do not treat babies without professional advice
(see also "Essential Oil Safety Precautions" - pages 17 & 18).

Also for highly odoriferous essential oils
Mix the essential oils to a 1/2 per cent dilution:
1 drop essential oil per 2 teaspoons (10 ml) essential oil.

QUICK GUIDE TO CARRIER OILS

A select list of popular carrier oils commonly used for aromatherapy massage and skin-care treatments.

Almond Oil (sweet) — Extracted from sweet, ripe almonds. Available both as a refined and unrefined oil. Has a light texture and high penetrative qualities. The most versatile carrier oil for massage or skin-care. Suitable for all skin types, including sensitive.

Apricot Kernel Oil — A refined oil extracted from the kernels ('stones') found in the fruit. A light textured oil used mainly in facial treatments and as a pre-wash conditioning treatment for dry hair. Good for mature, dry and sensitive skin.

Avocado Oil — Extracted from the flesh of the avocado. The unrefined oil is dark green, viscous and rich, yet highly penetrative. The refined version is pale yellow with little odour and fewer nutrients. Unrefined avocado oil is rich in vitamins A and E and lecithin. It also contains as yet unidentified substances that have been show to help regenerate skin cells. Avocado oil (refined or unrefined) is used mainly in facial treatments. May be used in combination with a light-textured oil such as sweet almond or grapeseed.

Grapeseed Oil — Available only in refined form. An extremely light-textured oil with a faint greenish hue. A popular aromatherapy base oil, due to its low odour.

Jojoba Oil — A natural liquid wax (commonly known as an 'oil') from the seeds of an evergreen desert plant. Naturally liquid at room temperature, becoming semi-solid in cooler conditions and having very little odour. A light-textured, highly penetrative oil used mainly for skin-care - including oily skin as it helps to unclog pores.. Its natural antibacterial properties give it a long shelf-life. May be used in combination with a less expensive oil such as sweet almond.

Rosehip Seed Oil — Solvent extracted from the tiny seeds found in rosehips. A light-textured oil with low odour. Rich in essential fatty acids and renowned for its ability to promote tissue regeneration. Used mainly as a facial oil.

Sunflower Seed Oil — The unrefined oil is light-textured with a slight nutty aroma. The refined version has a low odour. Unrefined sunflower seed oil contains more nutrients, including essential fatty acids and vitamin E. A useful multi-purpose oil for massage and skin-care, suitable for all skin types.

Safflower Oil — Extracted from the tiny seeds of this thistle-like plant. The unrefined oil is rich in the omega-6 group of essential fatty acids and contains appreciable quantities of vitamin E. It has a golden colour and slightly nutty aroma. However, unrefined safflower oil is highly unstable and difficult to keep fresh, so must be stored in the fridge. The refined version contains fewer nutrients, though has a longer shelf-life.

AROMATHERAPY SKIN-CARE CHART

A select list of essential oils commonly used in aromatherapy facial treatments.

Skin Type:	Description:	Essential Oils:
Normal	Soft, smooth, finely textured. Few problems like spots and flakiness.	Chamomile (Roman or German), lavender, rose, neroli.
Dry	Close-textured, but can feel tight after washing with soap. May also flake and is predisposed to developing facial lines.	Chamomile (Roman or German), rose, sandalwood.
Oily	Has a characteristic shiny look, usually with large pores; Prone to developing blackheads and pimples.	Frankincense, lavender, rosemary
Combination	Chin, nose and forehead form an oily T-zone , whereas the skin around the eyes and on the cheeks and neck is dry.	Lavender, frankincense, geranium, rose
Sensitive	Can be any type, and may become sensitive from exposure to harsh soaps and cosmetic materials. Always carry out a 24-hour patch test before using any skin care product (see page 19). Use essential oils in very low concentration e.g. 1/2 per cent.	Chamomile (Roman or German), rose, lavender.
Broken Capillaries (thread veins)	Broken veins usually occur around the nostrils and across the cheeks. Can affect all skin types, though more common on fair, sensitive skin.	Chamomile (especially German), frankincense, rose
Mature	In need of nourishing and toning.	Frankincense, geranium, neroli, sandalwood, rose.

AROMATIC BATH

Essential oils can be added to the bath simply for pleasure, to aid restful sleep, to help skin problems, relieve muscular aches and pains, ease cold and 'flu symptoms, and much more. Add 4-8 drops of essential oil after the bath has been filled. Swish the water around to disperse the oil. If you add the essential oil while the water is running, much of the aromatic vapour will have evaporated before you get into the bath. If you have dry skin, you may wish to mix the essences with a couple of teaspoons of carrier oil.

FOOT/HAND BATH

This method can be used for skin complaints of the hands and feet. An aromatic footbath at the end of a tiring day can be as relaxing as soak in a full-size bath. Put 4-6 drops of the appropriate essential oil in a bowl of hand-hot water, agitate the water to disperse the oil. Soak hands or feet for about 15 minutes. Dry thoroughly and massage into the skin a little vegetable oil (or skin cream) containing a few drops of the same essential oil(s).

INHALATIONS

Dry Inhalation:

For mood enhancement or to aid clarity of thought for study purposes, put a few drops of an appropriate essential oil on a tissue or handkerchief and inhale at intervals as required. For example, you might choose rose to uplift your spirits when feeling downhearted, or the piercing scent of rosemary to ease mental fatigue. To help clear nasal congestion or blocked sinuses, inhale eucalyptus or tea tree to supplement the benefits of steam inhalations. For nervous indigestion, inhale peppermint oil every few minutes until you experience relief. A few drops of lavender sprinkled on your pillow will aid restful sleep.

Steam Inhalation:

A good decongestant treatment, helpful for respiratory ailments such as coughs, colds and 'flu. Pour about 500 ml of near-boiling water into a bowl and then add 2-4 drops of essential oil. The quantity of essential oil depends on Odour Intensity   of the chosen essential oil. Peppermint, for example, is extremely odoriferous and will make you catch your breath if you use too much. In order to trap the aromatic steam, cover the bowl and your head with a towel to form a 'tent' and inhale for about 5 minutes. Steam inhalations can be taken two or three times a day over a short period.

Facial Steam

The steam inhalation method can be used as a weekly deep cleansing facial. Afterwards, splash your face with plenty of cool water to close the pores and remove tissue wastes which have been drawn to the surface.

CONSIDERATIONS:

Avoid steam treatments if you have broken capillaries (thread veins) as the intense heat may exacerbate the condition. Avoid steam inhalations if you have asthma: concentrated steam may trigger an attack.

AROMATIC COMPRESSES

A valuable first-aid measure for such problems as muscular aches and pains, skin eruptions, swellings, bruises, menstrual cramps. The most useful essential oils here are lavender or chamomile (Roman or German), as they have a wide range of therapeutic properties. However, it is important to know when to apply a hot compress, and when to apply a cold compress.

Hot

Helpful for old injuries, muscular pain, toothache, boils and abscesses. They can reduce pain and congestion in internal organs and are therefore helpful for menstrual cramp.

To make a hot compress, add about 6 drops of essential oil to a bowl containing about 500 ml of water, as hot as you can comfortably bear. Place a small towel, or a piece of lint or cotton fabric, on top of the water. Wring out the excess and place the fabric over the area to be treated. Cover this with a piece of plastic clingfilm, then lightly bandage in place if necessary (for ankle or knee, for example). Leave in place until the compress has cooled to body temperature; renew at intervals as required.

Cold

These are for recent injuries such as sprains, bruises, swellings and inflammation, and for headaches and fever.

For a cold compress, use exactly the same method as above, but with very cold water. Leave in place until the compress warms to body temperature; renew at intervals as required.

VAPORISATION

This method can be used as a fumigant to purify the air when infectious illness is around. It can also be used to create a subtle mood-enhancing ambience in the home or workplace.

Although there are many ways to vaporise essential oils, including adding a few drops to a radiator humidifier or a water-filled plant mister, a purpose-designed vaporiser is far more effective. Many of these gadgets are powered by mains electricity and use gentle heat to vaporise the oils into the room. Battery operated vaporisers are also available. Most electric vaporisers require undiluted essential oils, though a few allow for the oils to be diluted in a little water. Of the latter variety, the 'aromastone' (a heavy ceramic object) is the best as it affords the option of using either neat or diluted essential oils. There is also the stream diffuser or nebulizer, containing an air pump which sprays a fine mist of unheated essential oil into the room.

However, such gadgets are much more expensive than ordinary electric vaporisers.

The essential oil 'burner' (a misnomer since oils should never be burned!) is the most popular choice. Most burners are earthenware with attractive shapes cut out of the sides to afford a free flow of air for the night-light candle which fits inside. A small dish fits over the heat source and is filled with water. Essential oils are added to the water which is gently heated by the flame. As the water evaporates, the room becomes permeated with fragrance.

Since electric Vaporising equipment does not pose a fire risk they are particularly suitable for the workplace, and certainly much safer than night-lights for use in the bedrooms of children and elderly people.

Generally, you will need between 6-15 drops of essential oil, depending on the Odour Intensity of individual oils used, the capacity of your particular Vaporising equipment and the purpose for which the oil is intended. For mood enhancement, less is certainly more. As a fumigant, however, a stronger brew is recommended. If in doubt, follow the manufacturer's instructions.

MOUTHWASHES AND GARGLES

Ideal for sore throats and mouth ulcers.

Put a teaspoonful of cider vinegar in a teacup, then add 2 drops of an appropriate essential oil (e.g. tea tree). Top up with warm water and swish around the mouth, or use as a gargle. Do not swallow.

NB Essential oils are reasonably soluble in cider vinegar, so it makes a good natural dispersant for water-based concoctions. Cider vinegar also happens to be a traditional folk remedy for sore throats.

AROMATHERAPY PERFUMES

Many essential oils and absolutes make delightful skin perfumes when used singly or blended with other essences (see The Art of Blending, Chapter 3). They may be used purely for pleasure or to complement other aromatherapy treatment for healing emotional disharmony.
Dilute the essential oils in a low odour base oil such as sweet almond or Jojoba. The usual quantity is between 10 and 20 drops of essential oil to 10 ml of base oil. The exact quantity will depend on the Odour Intensity of your chosen aromatics. Let your nose be your guide.

CAUTION

The quantity of essential oil used in perfume blends is very much higher than for massage oils. Always carry out a 24-hour patch test (see page 19). However, if you have sensitive skin it is advisable to avoid this method of use, though you could perhaps perfume the ends of your hair.

AROMATIC OINTMENTS AND SKIN CREAMS

Many aromatherapy enthusiasts make their own ointments, creams and lotions using such ingredients such as beeswax, distilled water and almond oil - though it can be very time consuming. For busy people, most aromatherapy suppliers carry a range of unperfumed base products suitable for 'doctoring' with essential oils.

Ointment

Useful for such conditions as cuts, grazes, insect bites and stings, athlete's foot, ringworm, cold sores and chilblains. Add up to 25 drops of essential oil to 30g of an unperfumed base ointment. To make a general purpose antiseptic ointment, for example, you will need 10 drops lavender, 10 drops tea tree, and 10 drops geranium. Put the ointment in a little sterilised glass pot, and stir in the essences with the handle of a teaspoon. The ointment will keep for up to 6 months if stored in a cool, dark place.

Skin Cream

For aromatherapy skin-care treatments.

To a 30g pot of unperfumed skin cream, add 4-8 drops of essential oil and stir well with the handle of a teaspoon. To help you ascertain the correct essential oils for your skin type, refer to the 'Aromatherapy Skin-Care Chart' on page 12.

Skin - Tonics

Aromatic skin tonics can also be used as gentle aftershave. Cider vinegar is included in the basic formula because it helps to restore the skin's natural acid mantle. This can become disturbed by overuse of harsh soaps and cosmetics, resulting in dry, flaky or irritated skin. Apply skin tonic using cotton wool after washing or shaving to leave your skin feeling fresh and invigorated. Or pour a little in the palm of your hand and use as a splash.

Put 1 teaspoonful of cider vinegar into a 50ml dark glass bottle. Then add 2-3 drops of essential oil suitable for your skin type (refer to the Aromatherapy Skin-Care Chart, page 12) and shake well. Top up with distilled water (available from pharmacies) and shake again. For very oily skin or acne, you could use a more astringent base such as witchazel. This could be made slightly less astringent by mixing 50/50 with distilled water. Store in a cool dark place for up to 4 weeks.

CAUTION

Do not use tap water as this goes off very quickly. It also contains chlorine which is not good for the skin. Bottled water may be used, although even this has a limited shelf-life when used in skin tonics, depending on how often the contents come into contact with the germs on your hands. Even the cleanest hands harbour bacteria!

HAIR TONICS

These are made the same way as skin tonics. Since these are aqueous rather than oily, there is no need to shampoo it out after a limited time. If used regularly (3-4 times a week), an essential oil hair tonic will improve the condition of your hair and will make it smell good. If you have oily hair, you may find that regular use of a hair tonic reduces over-secretion of sebum, and thus the need to shampoo quite so frequently.

Put 3 teaspoons cider vinegar in 300 ml dark glass bottle, then add 15 drops of essential oil suitable for your hair and scalp condition (see Hair and Scalp Tonics Chart below) and shake well. Top up with distilled water and shake again. Shake well each time before use.

HAIR AND SCALP TONICS

Hair Type	Essential Oils:
Normal	Chamomile (Roman or German), geranium, lavender, neroli, mandarin, petitgrain, rose
Dry	Chamomile (Roman or German), lavender, sandalwood, rose, ylang ylang
Oily	Bergamot FCF, cypress, frankincense, juniper berry, lavender, lemon, patchouli, rosemary, tea tree.
Dandruff	Cypress, lavender, patchouli, rosemary, tea tree, chamomile (Roman or German), geranium.

NB Remember to choose an anti-dandruff oil which is also suitable for the condition of your hair (i.e. 'normal', 'dry' or 'oily')

ESSENTIAL OIL SAFETY PRECAUTIONS

Essential oils are wonderful healing substances, but they are highly concentrated and can be potentially hazardous if missed. So before you begin to experiment with essential oils, do please read the safety guidelines given here.

* Keep bottles out of reach of children

- Unsupervised skin applications of essential oils on babies and young children is not recommended. It is safer to use plain almond oil for massage, and/or to vaporise low concentrations (2-3 drops) of appropriate oils according to need. For children over the age of 5, use half the usual adult concentration of essential oil. Where there is the slightest doubt, please seek the advice of a qualified aromatherapist.

17

* Certain oils are best avoided during pregnancy. Always check the Considerations note in the Essential Oil Profiles – chapter 5 for any contra-indications. Generally, use essential oils in the lowest recommended quantities. If in doubt, seek the advice of a qualified aromatherapist.

* Nursing mothers should use essential oils in the lowest recommended quantities, as strong aromas can cause sleeplessness and irritability in babies. If in doubt seek the advice of a qualified aromatherapist. Avoid jasmine absolute as it may inhibit milk production.

* People with epilepsy are advised to avoid the following oils: fennel, hyssop, rosemary, sage. There is a remote chance that these oils may provoke a seizure in people predisposed to the condition.

* Keep essential oils away from varnished surfaces as they may dissolve the coating.
* Keep essential oils away from the eyes. Should any seep in, rinse with plenty of water. If this does not work, half-fill an eye bath with sweet almond oil and bathe the eye. Oil is the best medium for diluting essential oils.

* Never take essential oils by mouth, rectum (suppository) or vagina (pessary or douche). Although such methods are advocated by French aromatherapy doctors and clinical aromatherapists, unsupervised self-treatment is potentially risky.

* Essential oils should always be diluted before applying to skin. However, tea tree and lavender are occasionally applied neat to treat spots, insect bites and minor burns.

• Avoid steam inhalations if you suffer from asthma. Concentrated steam may trigger an attack.

* Citrus oils, especially bergamot, increase the skin's sensitivity to ultra violet light, so don't use on the skin within 12 hours of exposure to sunlight (or a sunbed) as they can cause unsightly pigmentation. It is possible to obtain a rectified bergamot oil labelled 'Bergamot FCF' (see page 40) which is virtually free of photosensitising agents.

* Avoid prolonged use of the same oil (i.e. daily for more than three months) as there is a slight risk of developing a sensitivity to it. Take a two-month break before using the same oil again.

• If you suffer from sensitive skin, carry out a 24-hour patch test (page 19) before using any essential oil for the first time (see below). However, if you suffer from eczema, asthma, allergic rhinitis or food allergies, it is essential to seek the advice of a qualified aromatherapist before embarking on treatment with essential oils. It may even be necessary to avoid aromatherapy altogether, and perhaps consult a homoeopath or medical herbalist.

* If you are having homoeopathic treatment, do seek the advice of your homoeopath before embarking on aromatherapy. Most strongly aromatic substances have the potential to negate the effects of homoeopathic remedies, though peppermint and eucalyptus are cited as particularly likely to do so.

* Never use an essential oil about which you can find little or no information.

PATCH TEST FOR SENSITIVE SKIN

When using essential oils for the first time, it is advisable to carry out a patch test especially if you have sensitive skin or suffer from allergies. Mix 3 drops of the test essential oil in a teaspoonful of your chosen carrier oil (e.g. almond, sunflower). Or, if using a blend of essential oils (as is most common in aromatherapy), you will need to test the mixture as a whole. Rub a little of the oil in the crook of your arm, behind your ear or on the inside of your wrist (supersensitive spots). Leave uncovered and unwashed for 24 hours. If there is no redness or itching, the oil is safe for you to use.

Using this method it's also possible to test three essential oils (or blends) at the same time. But you will need to keep an accurate record of the oils used and where they were applied. For example, one test oil applied to the wrist, another behind the ear and another in the crook of the arm.

CHAPTER 3

THE ART OF BLENDING

Concocting sweet-smelling massage oils, skin creams, bath mixtures and mood-enhancing room scents is sheer joy! Indeed, the practice of blending essential oils can be as therapeutic for the blender as it is for the recipient of the aromatic prescription.

Of course, there's no reason why a single essential oil should not be used if it is indicated for your therapeutic needs (refer to the essential oil profiles explored in this book). However, aromatherapists usually blend two, three or more oils to create a multi-faceted blend tailored to the person's physical and emotional needs - including their aroma preference. True, an uninteresting or medicinal-smelling oil can work well as a basic antiseptic, but in order to address the all important emotional aspect of our being (emotional disharmony is a contributing factor in many illnesses), common sense tell us that the aroma must be perceived as pleasing.

Interestingly, we tend to be instinctively drawn to the essential oil (or blend of oils) which best suits our physical and emotional needs at a given time. For the same reason, we can also 'go off' certain aromas when we no longer need their particular properties. For instance, it is common for pre-menstrual women to be attracted to the warm, sweet fragrance of Roman chamomile, a mildly sedative oil which is also helpful for headaches, skin eruptions and insomnia - common symptoms of PMS. Yet the same oil may well be perceived as 'sweet and cloying' when it is no longer needed.

DEVELOPING YOUR BLENDING SKILLS

Unlike pharmaceutical drugs, which are composed of relatively few chemical compounds, nature's essential oils are highly complex substances. As mentioned earlier, a single oil may contain hundreds of biochemical components. For this reason, all essential oils have multiple properties: they also share many properties in common. So it's not too difficult to create a pleasant-smelling blend to address your physical and emotional needs.

First select an oil which best matches your symptoms (refer to Quick Guide to Essential Oils for Common Ailments Page 116), taking into account your aroma preferences. For example, you may be suffering from nervous tension and muscular pain. Lavender would be an excellent choice (if you like the aroma), perhaps blended with a little frankincense and neroli. If you are not keen on lavender, there are numerous other oils which can relax taut muscles and soothe the mind - for example, cedarwood, clary sage and chamomile. Any of these oils could form the basis of your blend, supported with other compatible oils. To help you choose oils which blend well together, refer to the blending advice included in each of the Aromatic Profiles in Chapter 5.

As you will discover, the possibilities are endless! Simply allow your intuitive sense of smell to take you where it will. Most aromatherapists continue to develop their blending skills in this way. If, however, you would prefer more structured advice, let's explore a few basic 'rules'.

PERFUME NOTES

In very simple terms, a 'well balanced' blend is composed of top notes, middle notes and base notes (refer to the chart below). The top notes are highly volatile; they do not last very long (citrus oils). The middle notes last a little longer and impart warmth and fullness to the blend (rose otto, marjoram, Roman chamomile). Then there are the heavy base notes (patchouli, vetiver, sandalwood), which have a profound influence on the blend. They are very long lasting, and at the same time they 'fix' other aromas. This means they slow down the evaporation rate of the top and middle notes, thus increasing the staying power of the aromatic blend.

Now, you can choose to ignore all this about perfume notes if you wish - indeed, many aromatherapists do. After all, the system was invented by a perfumer, not an aromatherapist. Take the base notes, for example. None of the oils in this group would be suitable used in a burner (or inhaled from a tissue) to promote mental alertness. To sharpen the mind, it's important to choose highly volatile oils with a piercing or refreshing quality. Good examples are lemon, peppermint, pine and rosemary (top and middle notes). It would be counterproductive to add a heavy base note like sandalwood or vetiver to such a blend, as these oils tend to lull the mind into a quiet reverie.

Even perfumers have been known to break the rules. A classic eau de cologne blend, for example, is totally devoid of base notes. It's composed mainly of highly volatile citrus oils with a hint of rosemary. True, it has no staying power, but then it's sole purpose is to give a swift embrace like a splash of cool water: to refresh, enliven and uplift.

Perfume Notes Chart

Base	Base - Middle	Middle	Middle – Top	Top
		Black Pepper		Bergamot
	Cedarwood	Cardomom		
		Roman Chamomile		
	Cinnamon Leaf		Clary Sage	
			Coriander	
Frankincense				
	Ginger		Geranium	Grapefruit
			Ho Leaf	
	Jasmine Abs.			
	Juniper Berry			
		Lavender		Lemon
	Linden Blossom		Lemongrass	Lime
		Myrtle	Sweet Marjoram	Mandarin
		Neroli		
				Orange
Patchouli		Palmarosa	Peppermint	
			Petitgrain	
			Scots Pine	
	Rose Otto	Rose Abs.	Rosemary	
Sandalwood			Spearmint	
Vetiver				
	Ylang Ylang			

Odour Intensity Chart

A select list of essential oils and absolutes which you may find useful for creative blending.

Very Low	Low	Medium	Medium – High	High	Very High
	Bergamot			Black Pepper	
	Cedarwood	Coriander		Roman Chamomile	Cardomom
				Clary Sage	Cinnamon Leaf
				Frankincense	
		Grapefruit		Geranium	Ginger
		Ho Leaf			
			Juniper Berry	Jasmine Abs.	
			Lavender	Lime	Lemongrass
			Lemon	Linden Blossom	
Mandarin			Sweet Marjoram		
			Myrtle		
		Neroli			
		Orange			
			Petitgrain		Palmarosa
			Scots Pine		Patchouli
					Peppermint
		Rose Absolute	Rosemary	Rose Otto	
Sandalwood					Spearmint
Tangerine					
					Vetiver
				Ylang Ylang	

Oils commonly used in blending

Name	Aroma	Note	Mood	Odour Intensity
Bergamot	Citrus medium sweet	Top	Uplifting refreshing	Low
Black pepper	Spicy / camphoraceous	Middle	Stimulating, warming	High
Cardomom	camphoraceous / sweet / Spicy	Middle	Warming, mental stimulant	Very high
Cedarwood (Virginian)	Woody / balsamic pencil like	Base to middle	Calming, warming, grounding, aphrodisiac	Low
Chamomile, Roman	Herbaceous / sweet/ apple-like	Middle	Warming, comforting, calming	High
Cinnamon leaf	Spicy/ hot/ sweet	Base to middle	Stimulating, warming, restorative, aphrodisiac	Very high
Clary sage	Herbaceous/ musky-amber	Middle to top	Relaxing, cooling	High
Coriander	Spicy/ sweet	Middle to top	Restorative, warming, mental stimulant, aphrodisiac	
Frankincense	Resinous/ camphoraceous/ balsamic	Base	Restorative yet calming, warming, uplifting	High
Geranium	Rosy / sweet herbaceous	Middle-top	uplifting, restorative, refreshing	High
Ginger	Spicy /hot/ woody	Base to middle	Stimulating, warming, aphrodisiac	Very high
Grapefruit	Citrus/ sweet	Top	Uplifting, refreshing	Medium
Ho Leaf	Rosy/ woody	Middle to top	Uplifting, comforting, warming	Medium
Jasmine Absolute	Floral/ musky/ sweet	Base to middle	Uplifting, warming, aphrodisiac	High
Juniper berry	Peppery/ woody/ turpentine-like	Base to middle	Restorative, clearing, aphrodisiac	Medium to high
Lavender	Herbaceous / floral	Middle	Calming, cooling, yet also restorative	Medium to high
Lemon	Citrus/ sharp	Top	Uplifting, refreshing	Medium to high
Lime	Citrus/ bitter	Top	Refreshing, invigorating	High
Lemongrass	Lemony / herbaceous	Top to Middle	Refreshing, restorative	Very high
Linden Blossom	Hay-like/ sweet	Base to middle	Calming, intoxicating	High
Mandarin	Citrus/ sweet	Top	Soothing, comforting, gently uplifting	Very low
Marjoram (sweet)	Herbaceous/ camphoraceous/ spicy	Top to Middle	Warming, comforting	Medium-high
Myrtle	Camphoraceous/balsamic/ floral	Middle	Uplifting, restorative	Medium-high
Neroli	Floral/ sweet / refreshing	Middle	Calming yet uplifting, restorative	Medium
Orange (sweet)	Citrus/ sweet	Top	Uplifting, warming	Medium
Palmarosa	Rosy /herbaceous	Middle	Refreshing, restorative	Very high

Name	Aroma	Note	Mood	Odour Intensity
Patchouli	Earthy/ musky/ sweet	Base	Stimulating (relaxing in very small quantities), restorative, aphrodisiac	Very high
Petitgrain	Herbaceous/ woody/ fresh	Top to Middle	Calming, cooling, uplifting	Medium-High
Pine, Scots	Woody/ balsamic /Camphoraceous	Top to Middle	Refreshing, restorative, invigorating	Medium-High
Rose Absolute	Rosy/ floral	Middle	Soothing, comforting, uplifting, aphrodisiac	Medium
Rose Otto	Rosy/ floral	Base to middle	Soothing, comforting, uplifting, aphrodisiac	High
Rosemary	Camphoraceous woody-balsamic	Top to Middle	Mental stimulant, restorative, refreshing	Medium-High
Sandalwood	Woody/ balsamic	Base	Soothing, relaxing, aphrodisiac	Low.
Spearmint	Minty/ sweet herbaceous	Top to Middle	Refreshing, restorative	Very high
Tangerine	Citrus/ sweet	Top	Soothing, comforting, gently uplifting	Very low
Vetiver	Earthy/ sweet/ woody/ smoky	Base	Deeply relaxing, grounding	Very high
Ylang Ylang	Floral/ sweet/ balsamic	Base to middle	Uplifting, calming, aphrodisiac, intoxicating	High

HAPPY AROMA FAMILIES

It's always helpful to remember that 'families' of aromas generally blend harmoniously: herbaceous (clary sage/chamomile), citrus (bergamot/mandarin/ lemon), floral (rose/ neroli/ylang ylang), woody (cedarwood/sandalwood). Other compatible blends are spices with citrus (ginger/lemon/bergamot), florals with citrus (ylang ylang/lemon), peppery notes with woods (juniper berry/cedarwood), and resins with floral and citrus (frankincense/rose/mandarin). Woods and resins are good match too: frankincense/cedarwood is a classic. Oils from the fragrant grass family combine well, especially the lemony/floral scent of palmarosa with a hint of lemongrass.

You could also try marrying wildly differing personalities, such as the ancient and enigmatic frankincense with common or garden lavender; rose-scented geranium with a trace (no more!) of peppermint; heady neroli with a hint of musky patchouli or earthy vetiver. Another surprisingly scentsational blend is intoxicating jasmine, awakened with a tinge of black pepper. Two good all-rounders are clary sage and petitgrain. Although rather uninteresting when used alone, they act as 'bridges' to connect highly volatile oils like bergamot and mandarin with deeply resonating oils like cedarwood and sandalwood.

Aesthetically speaking, one of the most difficult oils to blend is tea tree. Its strong, medicinal odour tends to overpower the aromas of most other essential oils. However, it is quite acceptable blended with larger amounts of citrus oils, especially lemon. But on no account mix tea tree with fennel - a wonderful example of a disharmonious relationship!

25

ODOUR INTENSITY OF ESSENTIAL OILS

As well as tea tree, other highly odoriferous oils explored in this book include celery, fennel, lemongrass, Melissa, palmarosa, patchouli, peppermint spearmint valerian and vetiver. When experimenting with such oils - say, to create a massage oil blend - begin by adding just a single drop to 25 ml of vegetable base oil. Develop the blend by adding other essential oils drop by drop, and smelling as you go, until you achieve a desirable blend. To help you determine which oils blend well together, refer to the Blending Advice note given in each of the essential oil profiles.

When using a highly odoriferous oil in applications other than for massage, such as baths, steam inhalations and compresses, it's advisable to use no more than a single drop, augmented with a few drops of another compatible oil.

CHAPTER 4

THERAPEUTIC AND AESTHETIC BLENDING

The information given on this chart demonstrates the basic principles of therapeutic blending. It highlights two important medicinal actions of six popular essential oils and demonstrates how these properties may be enhanced using other aroma-compatible oils with similar therapeutic properties. It is especially interesting to note that ylang ylang, for example, can be sedative to the nervous system, especially when blended with soothing oils such as sandalwood and mandarin. On the other hand, when ylang ylang is combined with restorative oils such as lemongrass and coriander, its warming properties come to the fore, making it a good choice for sluggish circulation. For further information on the therapeutic properties and aroma compatibility of a number of essential oils refer to the Aromatherapy Uses and Aesthetic Blending Guide for each oil profiled in Chapter 5.

Focus on popular oils

Essential Oil	Properties in Focus	Blends to Enhance Properties
Bergamot	Antidepressant, heals wounds.	Uplifting Vaporising blend (in approximately 30ml water): 3 drops bergamot, 2 drops lavender, 1 drop rosemary, 1 drop geranium. Wound-healing lotion: 25ml distilled water, 1 teaspoon cider vinegar, 4 drops bergamot, 2 drops lavender, 2 drops eucalyptus. Put vinegar into a dark glass bottle, add essential oils and shake well. Top up with water and shake again. Apply with damp cotton wool pads.
Juniper berry	Sedative, diuretic	Sedative bath blend: 1 drop juniper berry, 2 drops clary sage, 3 drops mandarin. Massage oil for minor fluid retention (e.g. PMS): 25ml sweet almond oil, 4 drops juniper berry, 2 drops celery seed, 4 drops geranium, 2 drops grapefruit.
Lavender	Sedative, anti-rheumatic	Sedative Vaporising blend (in approximately 30ml water): 3 drops lavender, 1 drop spearmint, 2 drops clary sage. Anti-rheumatic massage oil: 25ml sweet almond oil, 5 drops lavender, 2 drops sweet marjoram, 1 drop ginger, 2 drops lemon.
Rose otto	Antidepressant, anti-inflammatory	Anti-depressant bath blend: 2 drops rose otto, 1 drop lime, 2 drops petitgrain, 2 drops clary sage. Anti-inflammatory bath for sunburn: 50ml cider vinegar, 1 drop rose otto, 2 drops Roman chamomile, 3 drops lavender. Mix the essential oils with the cider vinegar, then add to a tepid bath.
Rosemary	Mental stimulant, anti-rheumatic	Mentally stimulating Vaporising blend (in approximately 30ml water): 2 drops rosemary, 1 drop cardamom, 3 drops lemon. Massage oil for rheumatism: 25ml sweet almond oil, 4 drops rosemary, 2 drops frankincense, 2 drops juniper berry, 4 drops lavender.
Ylang Ylang	Sedative, circulatory stimulant.	Sedative massage oil: 25ml sweet almond oil, 2 drops ylang ylang, 2 drops sandalwood, 4 drops mandarin. Massage oil for poor circulation: 25ml sweet almond oil, 2 drops ylang ylang, 2 drops petitgrain, 2 drops lemongrass, 4 drops coriander.

AT-A-GLANCE REFERENCE - HEALING EMOTIONAL DISHARMONY

This chart represents the <u>possibilities</u> for emotional healing and is based on the law of averages. Your own responses may be quite different, so always be guided by your sense of smell and allow it take you where it will. Your chosen oil(s) may be used in the bath, in a massage blend, a vaporiser or inhaled from a tissue.

Emotional State	Suggested Healing Aromas
Grief:	Rose, marjoram, frankincense, pine, cypress, sandalwood, spikenard, valerian, helichrysum, vetiver.
Shock: Sudden emotional trauma:	Lavender, lemon, basil, bergamot, clary sage, melissa, neroli, peppermint, petitgrain, rosemary, eucalyptus, myrtle, rose.
Acute Anger: Irritability and frustration	Bergamot (and other citrus oils), Basil, Clary sage, peppermint, lavender, mandarin, pine, Roman chamomile, geranium, petitgrain.
Deep-rooted anger and frustration:	Rose, cedarwood (Atlas or Virginian), cypress, frankincense, ylang ylang, helichrysum, marjoram, neroli, spikenard, sandalwood.
Mood Swings:	Bergamot, mandarin, Roman chamomile, frankincense, geranium, juniper berry, lavender, lemon, rose, sandalwood, ylang ylang.
Despondency, despair, pessimism Initial stages of healing process:	Lavender, spikenard, sandalwood, cedarwood (Atlas or Virginian), cistus, clary sage, frankincense, cypress.
Later stages of healing process:	Bergamot (and other citrus oils), Basil, coriander, geranium, neroli, lemongrass, rose, rosemary, ylang ylang.
Worry, nervous tension, restlessness	Bergamot (and other citrus oils), Basil, Roman chamomile, cedarwood (Atlas or Virginian), cypress, frankincense, lavender, neroli, petitgrain, clary sage, myrtle, sandalwood, geranium, rose.
Poor concentration	Peppermint, lavender, myrtle, basil, cardomom, coriander, cypress, eucalyptus, frankincense, lemon, lime, lemongrass, pine, rosemary.
Confusion and Indecision	Bergamot (and other citrus oils), basil, cypress, eucalyptus, frankincense, geranium, myrtle, pine, peppermint, rosemary.
Fearfulness	Frankincense, basil, cypress, cedarwood (Atlas or Virginian), juniper berry, marjoram, rose, sandalwood, vetiver, palmarosa, lemongrass, spikenard, lavender.
Emotionally induced loss of libido	Rose, ylang ylang, ginger, coriander, clary sage, sandalwood, patchouli, cardomom, neroli, black pepper, juniper berry, jasmine.

BLENDING FOR EMOTIONAL HEALING

The sample formulas given below may be helpful for the conditions listed on the chart on the previous page. Of course, not every blend will not be right for every individual. Most of the recipes will need to be adjusted to suit personal preferences and responses. Nevertheless, the information should serve as an intriguing starting point. But don't forget, a single essential oil can be used as a healing tool if its aroma speaks to your innermost being.

TIP: When using an aromatic blend for self-massage, gently apply the oil to the solar plexus region (where the ribs make a 'v' shape), the back of the neck and soles of the feet. According to most healers, these areas of the body are especially vulnerable to the effects of psychic distress. The oils may also be used in the bath, a vaporiser or inhaled from a tissue.

For emotional healing, use the essential oil concentrates (see recipes below) in the following applications and dilutions:

Bath: 4-6 drops concentrate.

Massage Oil: 8-10 drops of concentrate in 25ml base oil

Dry Inhalation: 1-2 drops of concentrate on a tissue, inhaled at intervals as required.

Vaporiser: 6 drops of concentrate in an average candle-heated burner. For electric models, follow manufacturer's instructions.

THE HEALING BLENDS

In order to create harmonious blends, not every oil included in each recipe is recommended specifically for the named emotional state. The 'Grief' blend, for example, contains clary sage and spearmint which are not listed on the chart for this condition. Such essences are combined with the 'specifics' to enhance the aesthetic quality of the blend. So there is always space for creativity. Once you have blended your selection of oils, allow the mixture to settle for 24 hours before using it for the first time. This will enable the different elements to meld into a well-balanced composition.

IMPORTANT: The recipes on the following pages are *concentrated* mixtures of essential oils which can be used in a variety of ways for emotional healing. When following the recipes, measure the specified amount of undiluted essential oil into a dark glass bottle and shake well (each bottle of essential oil should be equipped with an integral dropper cap). To dispense the aromatic concentrate, use a pipette or eye dropper (available from pharmacies). Or, fit the dark glass bottle with a clean dropper cap (suitable 5ml and 10ml dark glass bottles with dropper caps are available from most essential oil suppliers see page 125).

THE HEALING BLENDS - Reference Chart
NB. These are concentrated formulas. Please read the instructions for use (page 29).

Grief: A suggested blend	6 drops rose otto (or 8 drops rose absolute) 2 drops spikenard 6 drops frankincense 10 drops lavender 8 drops clary sage 1 drop (no more!) spearmint
Shock: **A suggested blend** NB: For acute emotional shock, inhale melissa from a tissue (or one of the other oils listed on the chart on page 28).	10 drops frankincense 10 drops lavender 5 drops petitgrain 5 drops neroli 5 drops juniper berry
Deep-rooted anger and frustration **A suggested blend** NB: For acute anger, inhale one of the recommended oils from a tissue (see chart on page 28)	6 drops ylang ylang 10 drops sandalwood 3 drops lemongrass 10 drops Virginian cedarwood 5 drops petitgrain 5 drops clary sage
Mood Swings: **A suggested blend**	6 drops frankincense 5 drops bergamot 5 drops lemon 8 drops mandarin 5 drops neroli 6 drops lavender
Despondency, despair, pessimism Recipe 1 Initial stages of healing process	15 drops lavender 1 drop cistus (or 2 drops maximum) 12 drops clary sage 4 drops sandalwood 3 drops Atlas cedarwood
Despondency, despair, pessimism Recipe 2 Later stages of healing process	5 drops basil 5 drops bergamot 5 drops orange 5 drops mandarin 5 drops grapefruit 5 drops lemon 3 drops lime 5 drops coriander
Worry, nervous tension, restlessness **A suggested blend**	8 drops lavender 8 drops myrtle 8 drops clary sage 5 drops sandalwood 5 drops Scots pine

Poor concentration: **A suggested blend**	8 drops spearmint 8 drops peppermint 10 drops myrtle 8 drops lime
Confusion and Indecision: **A suggested blend**	5 drops cypress 5 drops petitgrain 5 drops pine 5 drops rosemary 5 drops frankincense 10 drops lemon
Fearfulness : **A suggested blend**	10 drops frankincense 4 drops palmarosa (or rose otto) 4 drops juniper berry 8 drops lavender 8 drops petitgrain 4 drops lemongrass
Emotionally induced loss of libido: **A suggested blend**	10 drops orange 8 drops mandarin 4 drops neroli 6 drops jasmine absolute (or ylang ylang) 5 drops patchouli 1 drop ginger (optional)

Chapter 5

ESSENTIAL OIL PROFILES

BOTANICAL CLASSIFICATION

In this directory the essential oil yielding plants are arranged in alphabetical order according to their English names. The Latin or botanical names are also given. This is important because the common names of plants differ from one region to another, whereas the botanical names are recognised throughout the world. But how did the botanical names come to be established?

Centuries ago each plant was known by a long, descriptive sentence, which was unwieldy, to say the least! It was not until the Swedish naturalist, Linnaeus (1707-1778), undertook the monumental task of methodically naming and classifying the whole living world 'from buffaloes to buttercups', that the dual name system became permanently established. In 1757 he was ennobled as Karl von Linné in recognition of his great contribution to science.

In the botanist's filing system, the first name of a plant, which always begins with a capital letter, signifies the genus (plural: genera). The second, the specific name or species, starts with a small letter. A third, subspecies (abbreviated subsp.) name is used to distinguish geographical variation within a species e.g. Neroli _aurantium subsp. aurantium._ and Petitgrain_C. _aurantium_ subsp. _Aurantium._ A multiplication symbol (X) between the first two names indicates a hybrid between two species e.g. Citrus x paradisi.

Over and above the generic name and the species name, plants are classified according to their family name - perhaps the most important sub-division of plant classification when considering identification. Plant families are categorised according to their shared characteristics. With the exception of non-flowering plants such as fungi and ferns, in approximate order of importance, these are:

Flower type, size and colour   Fruit or seed structure
Leaf structure and shape   Leaf and stem arrangement
Root or rhizome structure

BOTANICAL NAME CHANGES

It should be mentioned that botanists frequently, in the light of further research, change the names of various plants. In such instances, the most recent botanical name is given first, the earlier version being given as a synonym. (Incidentally, sometimes common name synonyms are included to allay possible confusion. Melissa, for example, is better known as Lemon Balm.) Plant families are also occasionally renamed - for example, the Asteraceae family was formerly known as Compositae. In such instances, the older name is given in brackets.

A WORD ABOUT BOTANICAL GENERALISATIONS

It is erroneous to assume that all plants within the same botanical family share the same (or similar) medicinal properties. Members of the Apiaceae (Umbelliferae) family, for instance, all produce clusters of flowers whose overall shape resembles that of an umbrella. Within this vast family resides the nutritious carrot, the culinary herbs dill and coriander, along with lethal hemlock and fool's parsley. Likewise, the Asteraceae or daisy family includes the gentle healers calendula and chamomile, with their poisonous cousin wormwood.

ℰngelica Seed-

Angelica archangelica

Plant Family: Apiaceae (Umbelliferae)

Note   Middle to top
Odour Intensity   Very high

Description:
A stout hairy plant with a large fleshy rhizome, ferny leaves and umbels of white flowers. Angelica is native to Europe and Siberia.

The oil is extracted by steam distillation of the roots or seeds: the latter is safest for home use (see Considerations).
It is a pale yellow liquid which becomes dark amber as it ages. The aroma is rich and earthy with an herbaceous top note. The odour effect is generally perceived as comforting and 'grounding'. Angelica seed oil is earthy-herbaceous with fruity and spicy top notes. It is similar to that of Angelica root, except that it additionally emanates a warming more uplifting quality.

Aromatherapy Uses:
Both the seed and root oils are helpful for congested skin conditions, arthritis, rheumatism, gout, fluid retention, bronchitis, colds, coughs, flatulence, indigestion, migraine, delayed periods (especially if stress-related), nervous exhaustion and other stress-related states. The oil is reputedly helpful as a supportive remedy for the recovering alcoholic because of its detoxifying properties.

Angelica oil (whether from the root or seed) is highly odoriferous and will overpower your blends unless used sparingly. Both oils actually blend well together. They also harmonise with Coriander, Bergamot (and other citrus oils), Cedarwood, Frankincense, Patchouli, Clary Sage, Vetiver.

Suggested Vaporising Blend:
To help soothe the effects of prolonged stress, especially if accompanied by nervous indigestion: 1 drop Angelica root, 3 drops Bergamot, 2 drops Lemon, 2 drops Coriander. The same combination and quantity of oils can be dropped on to a handkerchief and inhaled as needed.

Considerations:
Never apply Angelica root oil to skin shortly before exposure to natural or simulated sunlight, as it is highly phototoxic and can trigger severe pigmentation. The oil extracted from the seed, however, is regarded as non-phototoxic. Angelica oil (root and seed) reputedly promotes menstruation, so avoid skin applications during pregnancy. Angelica oil (root and seed) is highly odoriferous, so use in low concentration. Angelica root oil is not recommended for unsupervised home use.

niseed -

Pimpinella anisum

Plant Family: Apiaceae (Umbelliferae)

Note   Top
Odour Intensity   Very high

Description:
A dainty white-flowered annual with feathery leaves. The small brown seeds or fruit are ribbed and roundish. Anise is native to Greece and Egypt, though now widely cultivated mainly in India and to a lesser extent in China, Mexico and Spain. 'China', however predominantly produces Illicium verum (Star Anise), a quite different oil.

The oil is extracted by steam distillation of the seeds. It is a colourless to pale yellow liquid with a warm, spicy-sweet aroma. The odour effect is generally perceived as warming and stimulating.

Aromatherapy Uses:
Not much used in external treatments (see Considerations). French aromatherapy doctors prescribe oral doses of the oil, primarily for digestive and respiratory ailments. Aromatherapists occasionally use the oil in massage blends to ease muscular and rheumatic pain.

Aesthetic Blending Guide:
Aniseed does not blend well with many oils, for it tends to mask other aromas. To lessen its sweetness, however, it can be mixed with a larger quantity of Lemon and/or Bergamot. Aniseed oil is highly odoriferous, so use sparingly.

Suggested Vaporising Blend:
An unusual mood-elevating blend for those who can appreciate the penetrating aroma of Aniseed: 1 or 2 drops Aniseed (no more!), 3 drops Bergamot, 3 drops Lemon.

Considerations:
Aniseed oil contains a large proportion of anethole, which is known to provoke skin reactions in some people. Avoid external applications if you have sensitive or inflamed skin. Always use in the lowest recommended concentrations. Not recommended for unsupervised home use.

asil -

Ocimum basilicum

Plant Family: Lamiaceae (Labiatae)

Note   Top to middle
Odour Intensity   High

Description:
A tender shrub with highly aromatic leaves, native to tropical Asia and the Middle East, but now cultivated world-wide as a culinary herb.

The oil is extracted by steam distillation of the flowering tops and leaves. It is a colourless to pale yellow liquid, having a light, fresh, sweet-spicy scent with a balsamic undertone. Its odour effect is at first enlivening, giving way to a warm, comforting sensation.

Aromatherapy Uses:
Muscular aches and pains, colds and 'flu, delayed menstruation, as an insect repellent, mental fatigue, nervous tension, anxiety, mild depression.

Aesthetic Blending Guide:
Basil blends well with Bergamot, Lime, Lemon, Clary Sage, Frankincense, Geranium, Lemongrass, Neroli, Orange, Palmarosa.

Suggested Vaporising Blend:
To facilitate clarity of thought: 3 drops Basil, 2 drops Lemon, 3 drops Bergamot.

Considerations:
There are many varieties of Basil, several of which can be highly irritant to skin. Generally, Basil should be used in the lowest recommended concentrations. To harness the oil's insect repellent properties higher quantities may be necessary, so choose the vaporiser method. Avoid skin applications during pregnancy.

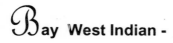# ℬay West Indian -

Pimenta racemosa

Synonym: Bay Rum

Plant Family: Myrtaceae

Note   Top
Odour Intensity   Medium

Description:
An evergreen tree with large leathery leaves and aromatic berries. The tree is native to the West Indies, particularly Dominica The oil is extracted by steam distillation of the leaves. It is light amber with spicy top notes, sweet middle notes and balsamic undertones. The odour effect is generally perceived as warming and stimulating.

Aromatherapy Uses:
Primarily used as a hair tonic to promote lustrous growth,   particularly for oily hair. Also helpful for dandruff, muscular aches and pains, neuralgia, rheumatic and arthritic pain, poor circulation, colds and 'flu, and as a fumigant when infectious illness is around.

Aesthetic Blending Guide:
West Indian Bay oil blends well with Bergamot (and other citrus oils), Coriander (and other spices), Geranium, Lavender, Lavandin, Rosemary, Ylang Ylang.

Suggested Hair Tonic Blend:
To help promote lustrous growth: 3 teaspoons cider vinegar (helps to maintain the natural acid/alkaline balance of the scalp), 2 drops West Indian Bay, 2 drops Ylang Ylang complete, 300 mls distilled water. Funnel the cider vinegar into a 300 ml dark glass bottle with a screw cap (available from pharmacies). Add the essential oil, then cover the opening with your thumb and give the bottle a good shake to disperse the oil droplets. Funnel the distilled water into the bottle and shake again.   Shake well each time before use. Apply 3-4 times a week to dry hair (i.e. not damp), massaging well into the scalp.   For convenience, you may prefer to funnel the tonic into a cosmetic spray bottle (preferably glass because essential oils may react with plastic if left in contact with the material for longer than a few weeks).   Store in a cool, dark place and use up within 6 weeks.

Considerations:
Do not use in steam inhalations as the oil may irritate the delicate mucous membranes in the upper part of the nose. Always use in the lowest recommended concentrations.

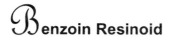enzoin Resinoid

Styrax tonkinensis

Plant Family: Styracaceae

Note   Base to middle
Odour Intensity   Low

Description:
A tender shrub with highly aromatic leaves, native to tropical Asia and the Middle East, but now cultivated world wide as a culinary herb.
Crude Benzoin is a balsamic resin obtained by making incisions in the bark of this large tree, native to tropical Asia. The resin hardens upon exposure to air and sunlight, forming Orange-brown 'tears' or 'pebbles'. These resin pieces are processed using solvents, for example benzene and alcohol, which are then evaporated off, leaving behind a reddish-brown viscous mass. This is usually sold dissolved in ethyl glycol (an alcohol) and labelled 'Benzoin Resinoid'. Although not an essential oil, Benzoin resinoid is commonly used in aromatherapy. It is an Orange-brown liquid with an intensely rich, sweet-balsamic aroma reminiscent of vanilla. Its odour effect is usually perceived as warming, soothing and comforting.

Aromatherapy Uses:
Inflamed skin, arthritic and rheumatic pain, gout, poor circulation, bronchitis, chills, coughs, laryngitis, colds and 'flu, nervous tension and other stress related states.

Aesthetic Blending Guide:
If using for massage, remember that Benzoin is only partially soluble in vegetable oil, so it is important to agitate the blend each time before use (i.e. by shaking the bottle of blended oil, or stirring the mixture if using a little bowl). Benzoin's main area of use is in steam inhalations (for respiratory ailments) and in vaporisers - as a fumigant or simply to perfume a room.   It blends well with Cedarwood, Ciste, Clary Sage, Sandalwood, Myrrh, Jasmine, Frankincense, Rose, Cypress, Pine, Juniper, Lemon, Coriander, Cinnamon, Ginger, Neroli, Cardomom, Clove, Ylang Ylang.

Suggested Vaporising Blend:
A deeply relaxing blend reminiscent of the sweet-resinous scent of amber: 3 drops Benzoin resinoid, 2 drops Clary Sage, 2 drops Sandalwood.

Considerations:
Although generally regarded as non-toxic and non-irritant, if used on the skin for prolonged periods (i.e. twice daily for upwards of 6 weeks) it may trigger sensitisation. Once sensitised, the skin will always react to any amount of the oil, no matter how tiny the quantity.   Never use 'Compound Benzoin' (also known as Friars Balsam) on the skin, as it is more likely to provoke sensitisation. It contains, in addition to Benzoin, storax, Tolu balsam, Aloe, and other substances. In this author's opinion, Benzoin resinoid extracted using the carcinogenic solvent benzene should be avoided. Although the amount present in the resulting product is negligible, this is beside the point. Benzene is detrimental to the health of people and the environment (distillery workers are at greatest risk) and therefore runs counter to the philosophy of holistic therapy. Always ask your supplier.

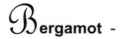# $\mathcal{B}$ergamot -

Citrus bergamia

Plant Family: Rutaceae

Note   Top
Odour Intensity   Low

Description:
Bergamots are the small, greenish-yellow, orange-like fruits of a small citrus tree. The primary world production centre is the Reggio di Calabria area of Italy, and then the Ivory Coast. It is the only citrus fruit grown and processed exclusively for its oil.

Interestingly this oil is most often associated with Sicily (a few kilometres away across the *Stretto di Messina*), but can not be *legally produced* there! The assumption that the oil is Sicilian arises from the large stocks of Italian Bergamot oil being held and distributed by local suppliers.

The oil is extracted by cold expression of the fresh peel of the fruit. It can be a green, red or yellow liquid with an aroma reminiscent of Orange and Grapefruit combined. Its odour effect is uplifting and refreshing.

Aromatherapy Uses:
Colds and flu, cystitis, fever, anxiety, mild depression, pre-menstrual tension.

Aesthetic Blending Guide:
Bergamot blends well with other citrus essences, also Angelica, Basil, Cedarwood, Chamomile (German and Roman), Clary Sage, Coriander, Lavender, Neroli, Cypress, Frankincense, Geranium, Ginger, Juniper, Lemongrass, Palmarosa, Petitgrain, Rose, Rosemary, Sandalwood, Vetiver.

Suggested Vaporising Blend:
For uplifting the spirits: 4 drops Bergamot, 2 drops Lemon, 2 drops Orange (sweet or bitter), 2 drops Neroli (or Petitgrain), 1 drop Rosemary.

Considerations:
The expressed oil is phototoxic because it contains high levels of furocoumarins. It should never be applied to skin shortly before exposure to natural or simulated sunlight (e.g. a sunbed) as it will cause unsightly pigmentation. However, from this author's experience, the oil can trigger the same skin reaction when applied shortly before exposure to hot, humid conditions such as a steamy hotel kitchen or laundry. For skin applications, Aromatherapists are increasingly using the rectified version known as Bergamot FCF (furocoumarin free), which is non-phototoxic. Whole Bergamot oil is best used solely as a mood-elevating room scent.

$\mathcal{B}$irch White -

Betula alba

Plant Family: Betulaceae

Note   Middle
Odour Intensity   Medium

Description:
A slender tree with silvery-white bark and pale green oval-shaped leaves. The tree is native to the cooler regions of Europe, northern China and Japan.

The oil is extracted by steam distillation of the leaf buds. It is a pale yellow, viscous liquid with a woody-balsamic aroma. The odour effect is generally regarded as cooling and invigorating. An oil is also produced by destructive distillation (the distillate is allowed to burn) of the bark: this is subsequently steam-distilled to produce rectified birch tar oil.

Aromatherapy Uses:
White Birch oil is helpful for skin and hair care (oily), cellulite, eczema (but only under the supervision of a clinical aromatherapist), muscular aches and pains, arthritic and rheumatic pain, poor circulation, fluid retention. Rectified birch tar oil is not generally used in aromatherapy, but forms the basis of pharmaceutical preparations (ointments, lotions and shampoos) for treating psoriasis.

Aesthetic Blending Guide:
White Birch oil blends well with Sandalwood, Cedarwood, Cypress, Frankincense, Pine, Rosemary.

Suggested Massage Blend:
To ease arthritic and rheumatic pain: 15 ml extra virgin Olive oil, 10 ml infused (macerated) St John's Wort oil, 5 drops White Birch, 4 drops Frankincense, 4 drops Rosemary.

Considerations:
Sensible precautions apply as with all concentrated essential oils. Refer to Essential Oil Safety Precautions pages 17 and 18.

$\mathcal{B}$lack $\mathcal{P}$epper

Piper nigrum

Plant Family: Piperaceae

Note   Middle
Odour Intensity   High

Description:
A large twining plant or vine, native to India, but now extensively cultivated in Malaysia, China and Madagascar. India however, still remains the single largest source for the oil.

The oil is extracted by steam distillation of the dried fruits (Peppercorns). It is a pale, greenish-yellow liquid, with a hot, spicy, piquant aroma. Its odour effect is stimulating and warming: a reputed aphrodisiac.

Aromatherapy Uses:
Poor circulation, muscular aches and pains, loss of appetite, nausea, colds and 'flu, lethargy, mental fatigue.

Aesthetic Blending Guide:
Black Pepper blends well with other spices, citrus essences, Frankincense, Jasmine, Lavender, Geranium, Rose, Ylang Ylang, Rosemary, Sandalwood.

Suggested Massage Oil Blend:
For soothing aching muscles: it also makes a warming aphrodisiac blend! 25 ml vegetable base oil, 3 drops Jasmine, 3 drops Coriander, 2 drops Black Pepper.

Considerations:
For skin applications, use in the lowest recommended concentrations. Applications of the oil are best avoided during the first trimester of pregnancy.

ajuput -   *Melaleuca leucadendron*

Plant Family: Myrtaceae

Note   Top
Odour Intensity   Medium to high

Description:
A tall evergreen tree with slender leaves, white flowers and a whitish spongy bark which flakes off easily. Cajuput is native to Malaysia, Indonesia, the Philippines, Australia and south-eastern Asia.

The oil is extracted by steam distillation of the leaves, buds. It is a pale yellow liquid with a camphoraceous, slightly Peppery aroma. Its odour effect is head-clearing and stimulating.

Aromatherapy Uses:
Acne, insect bites and stings, arthritis, muscular aches and pains, rheumatism, stiff joints, bronchitis, catarrh, coughs, sinusitis, sore throat, cystitis, colds and 'flu, as a fumigant when infectious illness is around.

Aesthetic Blending:
Like other oils of the Melaleuca family (e.g. Tea Tree, Niaouli), Cajuput does not blend very well with other essential oils. However, it is acceptable mixed with Bergamot, Lemon, Lavender, Lavandin, Rosemary, Juniper, Cypress, Pine. The oil is highly odoriferous and will overpower your blends unless used sparingly.

Suggested Steam Inhalation Blend:
For easing cold and 'flu symptoms, catarrh, sinusitis and other minor respiratory infections: pour about 2 pints of steaming water into a large, heatproof bowl. Add 2 drops Cajuput and 2 drops Lavender. Put a towel over your head and the bowl to form a 'tent' and inhale the aromatic vapours for 5 minutes.

Considerations:
Cajuput oil has been reported to cause skin irritation. However, the chance of this occurring is greatly reduced if the rectified oil is used. Many of the problems associated with Cajuput may also be due to the fact that it is often adulterated with substances such as turpentine (highly irritant to skin) and synthetic colourant. It is essential to obtain the oil from a reputable supplier who can vouch for its purity.

Camphor - White -

Cinnamomum camphora

Plant Family: Lauraceae

Note   Top
Odour Intensity   Very high

Description:
A tall evergreen tree bearing clusters of small white flowers and red berries. It produces a white crystalline substance, the crude camphor, from the wood of mature trees over fifty years old. The tree is native to Japan and China, though cultivated in other regions such as Egypt, Madagascar and the USA.

The oil is extracted by steam distillation of the wood. Before the oil can be used therapeutically, it has to be re-distilled or rectified. This produces three grades (fractions), known as White, Brown and Yellow Camphor. Only White Camphor is considered safe for aromatherapy (see Considerations). The oil is a colourless to pale yellow liquid with a strong, sharp, camphoraceous odour. Its odour effect is head-clearing: a reputed anaphrodisiac (quells sexual desire).

Aromatherapy Uses:
Not much used in aromatherapy because of its overpowering medicinal aroma. However, it can be helpful for acne, muscular aches and pains, arthritic and rheumatic pain, sprains, as an insect repellent, bronchitis, coughs, colds and 'flu, as a fumigant when infectious illness is around.

Aesthetic Blending Guide:
 A difficult oil to blend, for its pungent odour tends to overpower the aromas of other essential oils. However, its camphoraceous quality can be lessened somewhat by mixing with a larger quantity of Lemon oil. Alternatively, try sweetening the aroma by blending with Ho leaf oil (extracted from the leaves of a closely related tree) and/or Palmarosa.

Suggested Vaporising Blend:
Use as a fumigant when infectious illness is around: 4 drops White Camphor, 3 drops Ho-leaf, 3 drops Palmarosa.

Considerations:
Brown and yellow Camphor contain dangerously high levels of saffrol (a carcinogenic agent) and should never be used for aromatherapy. Although White Camphor is considered to be non-toxic and non-irritant, it is advisable to use the oil in the lowest recommended concentrations as it is highly odoriferous. It is also best suited to local applications and inhalations, rather than full-body treatments. Avoid during pregnancy: do not use on babies and young children.

$\mathcal{C}$araway -   *Carum carvi*

Plant Family: Apiaceae (Umbelliferae)

Note   Middle
Odour Intensity   High

Description:
A biennial herb with feathery leaves and umbels of white flowers. The small dark seeds or fruit are carved with five distinct pale ridges. Caraway is native to Europe and western Asia.

The oil is extracted by steam distillation of the dried seed or fruit. It is a pale yellow liquid which darkens as the oil matures. The aroma is hot, sweet and spicy with fruity nuances. Its odour effect is warming and stimulating.

Aromatherapy Uses:
Colds and 'flu, bronchitis, coughs, nervous indigestion, colic, flatulence, scabies. Reputedly promotes menstruation, but it may need to be taken internally for this purpose - a potentially risky method for the home user. If the aroma is liked, it can also be helpful for nervous exhaustion.

Aesthetic Blending Guide:
Caraway is highly odoriferous and will overpower your blends unless used with discretion. Try a tiny amount with Coriander, Cinnamon, Black Pepper, Cardomom, Lemon, Jasmine, Geranium.

Suggested Vaporising Blend:
A rich, spicy-floral blend to warm the soul on a cold winter's night: 2 drops Caraway, 3 drops Coriander, 2 drops Jasmine.

Considerations:
The oil can be irritant to skin unless used in low concentrations of 1 % (i.e. 1 drop per 5 ml base oil) or less. Best avoided during pregnancy as it reputedly stimulates menstruation.

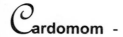ardomom -

Elettaria cardomomum

Plant Family: Zingiberaceae

Note   Middle
Odour Intensity   Very high

Description:
A reed-like plant with yellowish flowers, producing reddish-brown seeds or fruit. While Cardomom is native to tropical Asia and especially southern India, the predominant production area is Central America.

The oil is extracted by steam distillation of dried fruit or seeds. It is a colourless to pale yellow liquid. The aroma is sweet, spicy and balsamic with a hint of Eucalyptus. It's odour effect is warming, head-clearing and enlivening: a reputed aphrodisiac.

Aromatherapy Uses:
Indigestion, colic, flatulence, offensive breath, mental fatigue, nervous exhaustion.

Aesthetic Blending Guide:
Cardomom blends well with Cedarwood, Frankincense, Caraway, Cinnamon, Cloves, Ginger, citrus oils, Ciste, Rose, Jasmine, Geranium, Lavender, Neroli, Ylang Ylang. The oil is highly odoriferous, so use sparingly.

Suggested Mouthwash Blend:
This mixture can be used after meals to sweeten the breath. 200 ml distilled water, 2 teaspoons cider vinegar, 1 drop Cardomom, 5 drops Coriander, 5 drops Bergamot FCF. Put the cider vinegar into a dark glass medicine bottle (available from pharmacies), then add the essential oils and shake well. Funnel the distilled water into the bottle. To use: add a few teaspoons of the mixture to a teacupful of warm water. Swish around the mouth, then spit it out. Repeat several times, or until the mixture is used up. Remember to shake the bottle each time before use to disperse the oil droplets.

Considerations:
Generally regarded as non-irritant and non-sensitising. Like most spice oils, however, it is powerful in its effect and must be used in low concentrations.

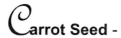arrot Seed -

Daucus carota

Plant Family: Apiaceae (Umbelliferae)

Note   Middle
Odour Intensity   Medium to high

Description:
A yellow or amber-coloured liquid with a warm, spicy, woody-earthy aroma. Its odour effect is warming and enlivening. Most of the oil is produced in France.

The oil is extracted by steam distillation of the dried seeds of wild carrots whose fibrous roots are inedible.

Aromatherapy Uses:
Eczema, psoriasis, general skin care (for revitalising and toning),
arthritis, rheumatism, gout, as a supportive remedy for detoxification purposes, as a restorative during convalescence, indigestion, liver congestion, pre-menstrual syndrome (especially to help with fluid retention).

Aesthetic Blending:
Carrot seed oil blends well with Bergamot (and other citrus oils), Coriander (and other spices), Cedarwood, Fennel, Roman Chamomile, Geranium, Lavender, Rose, Ylang Ylang.

Suggested Massage Oil Blend:
A beauty oil for toning and revitalising mature skin: 10 ml Rosehip carrier oil, 10 ml Sweet Almond carrier oil, 2 drops Carrot seed oil, 1 drop Rose Otto (or 2 drops Lavender).

Considerations:
Best avoided during the first trimester of pregnancy as the oil reputedly stimulates menstruation.

$\mathcal{C}$edarwood, Virginian -

Juniperus virginiana

Plant Family: Cupressaceae

Note   Middle to base
Odour Intensity   Low

Description:
An evergreen conifer tree native to eastern and central North America.

The oil is extracted by steam distillation of the wood, stumps and sawdust. It is a yellowish amber, viscous liquid with a sweet, woody aroma which improves as the oil ages. Its odour effect is gently head-clearing, grounding and calming: a reputed aphrodisiac.

Aromatherapy Uses:
Acne, oily skin, dandruff, fungal infections, arthritis, rheumatism, respiratory ailments, pre-menstrual syndrome, loss of menstruation outside pregnancy, nervous tension, stress-related disorders.

Aesthetic Blending Guide:
Cedarwood blends well with Benzoin, Bergamot, Clary Sage, Cypress, Frankincense, Geranium, Jasmine, Juniper berry, Lemon, Neroli, Mimosa, Palmarosa, Petitgrain, Pine, Rose, Rosemary, Sandalwood, Vetiver, Ylang Ylang.

Suggested Massage Oil Blend:
For rheumatic aches and pains: 25 ml vegetable base oil, 5 drops Cedarwood, 2 drops Cypress, 2 drops Juniper berry, 2 drops Lemon.

Considerations:
Avoid during pregnancy. The oil may irritate sensitive skin: use in the lowest recommended concentrations.

*C*elery Seed -

Apium graveolens

Plant Family: Apiaceae (Umbelliferae)

Note   Middle
Odour Intensity   High

Description:
A biennial plant with a grooved, fleshy, erect stalk, feathery leaves and umbels of white flowers. The small seeds are greyish brown. Celery is native to southern Europe, though extensively cultivated throughout the world.

The oil is captured by steam distillation of the whole or crushed seeds. It is a pale yellow liquid with a sweet, tenacious aroma, characteristically Celery. The odour effect is restorative and calming: a reputed aphrodisiac.

Aromatherapy Uses:
Arthritis, rheumatism, gout, as a supportive remedy for detoxification purposes, chilblains, cystitis, indigestion, flatulence, liver congestion, loss of periods outside of pregnancy, to increase milk flow, neuralgia, sciatica, pre-menstrual syndrome (especially to help reduce fluid retention), nervous exhaustion.

Aesthetic Blending Guide:
Celery seed oil is very tenacious with a powerful and distinctive aroma. If used sparingly, it mixes well with Coriander (and other spices), Clary Sage, Lavender, Pine.

Suggested Bath Oil Blend:
For nervous exhaustion: 2 drops Celery seed, 3 drops Clary Sage, 2 drops Lavender.

Considerations:
The oil is highly odoriferous, so use in the lowest recommended concentrations. Avoid during pregnancy.

Chamomile, German - *Matricaria recutica*

Synonym: *Matricaria chamomilla*

Plant Family: Asteraceae (Compositae)

Note   Middle
Odour Intensity High

Description:
A strongly aromatic herb with delicate feathery leaves and simple daisy-like white flowers. The plant is native to Europe and north and west Asia.

The oil is captured by steam distillation of the flower heads. An inky-blue, viscous liquid with a sweetish, warm-herbaceous aroma. Its odour effect is gently warming and soothing.

Aromatherapy Uses:
Skin care (most skin types including sensitive), eczema (but see Considerations below), skin rashes, boils, burns, wounds, chilblains, earache, insect bites and stings, inflammation and swelling (e.g. caused by injury), muscular aches and pains, arthritic and rheumatic pain, sprains and strains, neuralgia, teething pain, toothache, indigestion, painful periods, heavy periods, headache, migraine, insomnia, pre-menstrual syndrome, nervous tension, and other stress-related states.

Aesthetic Blending Guide:
German Chamomile blends well with Bergamot (and other citrus oils), Rose, Lavender, Geranium, Neroli, Marjoram, Clary Sage, cistus, Ylang Ylang.

Suggested Skin Cream Blend:
Soothes skin rashes and patches of dry eczema: 15g unperfumed base cream (available from aromatherapy suppliers), 5 ml macerated Calendula oil, 6 drops German Chamomile. Mix the Calendula oil into the base cream with the handle of a teaspoon, then stir in the essential oil. Apply 3 times a day. Store the cream in a cool dark place and use up within 4 weeks.

Considerations:
Although German Chamomile oil is helpful for allergic skin reactions, it must always be used in the lowest recommended concentrations, otherwise it may actually exacerbate the condition. When treating chronic eczema it is essential to seek the advice of an holistic practitioner, such as a clinical aromatherapist, medical herbalist or nutrition counsellor, who will be able to devise a personalised treatment programme to address the underlying cause of the condition.

$\mathcal{C}$hamomile, Maroc -   *Ormenis multicaulis*

Synonym: Ormensis Flower

Plant Family: Asteraceae (Compositae)

Note   Middle
Odour Intensity   High

Description:
An attractive plant with hairy leaves and tubular, yellow flowers.

The oil is extracted by steam distillation of the flowering tops. It is a yellow to light amber liquid with a sweet, herbaceous aroma somewhat akin to Roman Chamomile. Its odour effect is generally perceived as soothing.

Aromatherapy Uses:
Little is known about the oil's therapeutic history as it's a relative newcomer to aromatherapy (see also Considerations). Preliminary findings have shown it to be helpful for headache, insomnia, painful periods, and as a mood-enhancing room scent for reducing stress.

Aesthetic Blending Guide:
Chamomile Maroc blends well with Cedarwood, Clary Sage, Lavender, Lavandin, Lemon, Ciste, Cypress, Petitgrain, Frankincense.

Suggested Vaporiser Blend:
A soothing formula for reducing stress and anxiety: 3 drops Chamomile Maroc, 3 drops Petitgrain, 2 drops Frankincense.

Considerations:
Although generally regarded as non-toxic and non-irritant, more specific safety data is unavailable at present. For this reason, it's best used in the lowest recommended concentrations. Skin applications should be avoided by pregnant women and anyone with sensitive skin.

Chamomile, Roman -

Chamaemelum nobile

Plant Family:

Asteraceae (Compositae)

Note   Middle
Odour Intensity High

Description:
A small, stocky herb with feathery leaves and daisy-like white flowers. The plant is native to Europe and North America.

The oil is extracted by steam distillation of the flower heads. It is a pale yellow liquid with a sweet aroma reminiscent of ripe apples. The odour effect is warming and calming.

Aromatherapy Uses:
Skin care (most skin-types), acne, eczema, inflamed skin conditions, earache, wounds, menstrual pain, pre-menstrual syndrome, headache, insomnia, nervous tension and other stress-related disorders.

Aesthetic Blending Guide:
Roman Chamomile blends well with citrus essences, Clary Sage, Lavender, Geranium, Jasmine, Neroli, Rose. The oil is highly odoriferous, so use sparingly in blends.

Suggested Aromatic Bath:
To promote restful sleep: 3 drops Roman Chamomile, 2 drops Clary Sage, 1 drop Lavender.

Considerations:
Avoid skin applications during the first trimester of pregnancy. May cause skin irritation in susceptible individuals. The oil is highly odoriferous, so use in the lowest recommended concentrations. Due to the high price of Roman Chamomile, there is a tendency for some essential oil suppliers to promote Moroccan Chamomile (*Ormensis multicaulis*) as a cheaper alternative. Although the plant is distantly related to Roman Chamomile and has a similar aroma, its medicinal properties have not been thoroughly investigated.

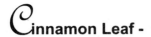innamon Leaf -

Cinnamomum zeylanicum

Plant Family: Lauraceae

Note   Base to middle
Odour Intensity   Very high

Description:
Cinnamon is a tree native to Sri Lanka and Southern India, but cultivated in many other tropical regions for the spice trade.

The oil is extracted by steam distillation of the leaves and twigs. It is a yellowish liquid with a pungent, warm-spicy, somewhat harsh aroma. The oil extracted from the bark has a superior aroma, but unfortunately it is unsuitable for aromatherapy (see Considerations). The odour effect of Cinnamon is warming and enlivening.

Aromatherapy Uses:
Poor circulation, rheumatism, indigestion, delayed periods outside pregnancy, colds and 'flu, nervous exhaustion.

Aesthetic Blending Guide:
Cinnamon leaf blends well with Benzoin, citrus essences, Coriander, Frankincense, Ylang Ylang. However, it must be used in tiny quantities, otherwise its powerful aroma will predominate your blends.

Suggested Vaporising Blend:
A warming, heady Oriental blend, especially delightful on a cold winter's night: 1 drop Cinnamon leaf, 5 drops Orange, 2 drops Benzoin, 1 drop Ylang Ylang.

Considerations:
Avoid skin applications during pregnancy. Cinnamon leaf oil should never be used on sensitive skin as it can be highly irritant. For aromatherapy massage, it is advisable to use in the lowest recommended concentrations of around 0.5%, perhaps blended with other suitable essences according to aroma compatibility and therapeutic requirement. It is advisable to avoid using the oil in the bath or in steam inhalations because heat and humidity increase its tendency to irritate skin and mucous membranes. However, the oil can be vaporised as a fumigant (with other essences if desired) when infectious illness is around. Cinnamon bark oil is classified as a dermal toxin, irritant and sensitiser and must never be used on the skin.

$\mathcal{C}$iste -

Cistus ladaniferus

Synonyms: Cistus, labdanum,
                 Rock Rose.

Plant Family: Cistaceae

Note   Base
Odour Intensity Extremely high

Description:
Ciste is a small, sticky shrub with lance-shaped leaves and fragrant white flowers native to the Mediterranean and Middle East.

The oil is extracted by steam distillation of the crude gum (an oleoresin obtained by boiling the leaves and twigs in water). Moreover, an essential oil can be obtained by distilling the plant material directly. A solvent extracted absolute is also available. The absolute is a semi-solid, dark green mass with a rich, sweet and balsamic aroma. The essential oil (whether extracted from the oleoresin or from the leaves and twigs directly) is a light amber liquid with a very strong, sweet, dry-herbaceous, musky aroma. Its odour effect is warming, stimulating and uplifting: a reputed aphrodisiac.

Aromatherapy Uses:
Skin care (especially mature), bedsores, infected wounds, skin ulcers, bronchitis, coughs, colds and 'flu, as a fumigant when infectious illness is around, absence of periods outside pregnancy, vaporised as a meditation aid.
Although some authorities describe Ciste as a relaxant, this may well be a reference to the gentler quality of the absolute. In this author's experience, the oil is undoubtedly stimulating and restorative. An excellent oil to use during convalescence or when suffering from nervous exhaustion.

Aesthetic Blending Guide:
Ciste blends well with Angelica, Cedarwood, Coriander, Chamomile Maroc, Clary Sage, Cypress, Lavender, Lavandin, Frankincense, Jasmine, Juniper, Pine, Rose, Lemon (and other citrus oils), Neroli, Petitgrain, Sandalwood, Patchouli, Vetiver. However, the oil is highly odoriferous and will overpower your blends unless used very sparingly.

Suggested Massage Blend:
A wonderful restorative formula for nervous exhaustion and mild depression: 30 ml vegetable base oil, 1 drop Ciste, 3 drops Scots Pine, 3 drops Frankincense, 3 drops Petitgrain, 5 drops Bergamot FCF. If you really think you can take it, add an extra drop of Ciste - certainly no more!

Considerations:
Avoid during pregnancy. Best used in low concentrations, as it can be over-stimulating.

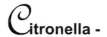

Citronella -

Cymbopogon nardus

Plant Family: Poaceae (Gramineae)

Note   Top
Odour Intensity   Very high

Description:
Citronella is an aromatic grass native to Sri Lanka.

The oil is extracted by steam distillation of the fresh or dried grass. It is a virtually colourless liquid with a strong, sweet, woody-Lemony aroma. The scent is similar to Lemongrass, although harsher and even more odoriferous. Its odour effect is cooling and enlivening.

Aromatherapy Uses:
Insect repellent, colds and 'flu (and other feverish conditions), headaches, migraine, rheumatic pain. Some authorities recommend the oil for skin care (oily skin). However, in this author's opinion the oil is far too strong for such purposes (see Considerations).

Aesthetic Blending Guide:
Citronella does not blend very well with other oils because of its overpowering aroma. If used sparingly, however, it is acceptable mixed with Cedarwood, Geranium, Palmarosa, Pine.

Suggested Vaporising Blend:
To repel flies: 2 drops Citronella, 3 drops Geranium, 3 drops Cedarwood.

Considerations:
Avoid during pregnancy as the oil reputedly stimulates menstruation. It may also irritate sensitive skin.

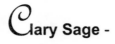 **lary Sage -**   *Salvia sclarea*

Plant Family: Lamiaceae (Labiatae)

Note   Middle to top
Odour Intensity   High

Description:
Clary sage is a shrubby, highly aromatic herb with spikes of white, violet or pink flowers. It is native to the Mediterranean.

The oil is extracted by steam distillation of the flowering tops and leaves. It is a colourless to pale yellow liquid. The aroma of a good quality oil is sweetly herbaceous with a floral tinge. Its odour effect is uplifting and relaxing: a reputed aphrodisiac.

Aromatherapy Uses:
High blood pressure, muscular aches and pains, respiratory ailments, migraine, to facilitate childbirth, irregular menstruation, pre-menstrual syndrome, menopausal distress, mild depression, nervous tension and other stress-related states.

Aesthetic Blending Guide:
Clary Sage blends well with most oils, especially Benzoin, Bergamot, Cedarwood, Jasmine, Mimosa, Juniper berry, Lavender, Neroli, Petitgrain, Pine, Frankincense, Vetiver.

Suggested Massage Oil Blend:
To help alleviate nervous tension and anxiety: 25 ml of vegetable base oil, 3 drops Clary Sage, 3 drops Bergamot FCF, 3 drops Cedarwood.

Considerations:
Avoid skin applications during pregnancy. Although the oil is commonly believed to cause excessive drowsiness when used immediately before or after drinking alcohol, Clary may not be especially potent in this respect. In this author's experience <u>any</u> form of relaxing massage (with or without sedative or heady essential oils) will intensify the effects of alcohol.

$\mathcal{C}$love -

Syzgium aromaticum

Synonyms: Eugenia caryophyllus,
                                                   E. Caryophyllata

Plant Family: Myrtaceae

Note   Middle
Odour Intensity   Extremely high

Description:
A slender evergreen tree with brilliant red flowers. When dried the flower buds turn reddish-brown.   The tree is believed to be native to Indonesia, but is cultivated extensively in other tropical regions.

There are three grades of steam distilled Clove oil: Clove bud, Clove leaf and Clove stem. The best grade for aromatherapy is Clove bud (but see Considerations). Clove bud oil is a pale amber liquid with a strong, sweet-spicy, fruity aroma. The other two grades of Clove oil have much harsher aromas. Clove oil's odour effect is generally perceived as warming and stimulating: a reputed aphrodisiac.

Aromatherapy Uses:
Although some aromatherapists use low concentrations of Clove bud oil on the skin for conditions such as acne, athlete's foot and as an insect repellent, this is not recommended for unsupervised home use (see Considerations). However, the oil can be used in a vaporiser as a room scent or fumigant, or as a first-aid measure for toothache (a single drop in the tooth cavity or massaged into the gum) while awaiting dental treatment.

Aesthetic Blending Guide:
Clove oil blends well with citrus oils, Frankincense, Geranium, Lavender, other spices, Rose, Ylang Ylang. The oil is highly odoriferous and will overpower your blends unless used very sparingly.

Suggested Vaporising Blend:
A warming and uplifting room scent: 1 drop Clove oil, 2 drops Lavender, 5 drops Orange.

Considerations:
All three grades of Clove oil are very irritant to skin and mucous membranes because they contain high amounts of eugenol (a caustic biochemical). Clove leaf and Clove stem oils contain even greater amounts of the substance. Use with utmost caution, preferably only as a Vaporising oil. Avoid during pregnancy.

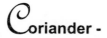oriander -

Coriandrum sativum

Plant Family: Apiaceae (Umbelliferae)

Note   Middle
Odour Intensity   Medium

Description:
A strongly aromatic herb with bright green delicate leaves and umbels of lace-like white flowers, followed by a mass of green (turning brown) seeds or fruit. Coriander is native to Europe and western Asia.

The oil is extracted by steam distillation of the crushed, ripe seeds. It is a colourless to pale yellow liquid with a pungent, sweet-spicy, faintly musky aroma. Its odour effect is warming, uplifting and stimulating: a reputed aphrodisiac.

Aromatherapy Uses:
Arthritic and rheumatic pain, muscular aches and pains, facial neuralgia, poor circulation, digestive problems, colds and 'flu, mental fatigue, nervous exhaustion.

Aesthetic Blending Guide:
Coriander blends well with other spices, Ciste, citrus oils, Geranium, Rose, Cypress, Jasmine, Juniper, Petitgrain, Neroli, Pine, Frankincense, Sandalwood.

Suggested Bath Blend:
A warming, restorative blend for nervous exhaustion: 3 drops Coriander, 1 drop Ciste, 2 drops Orange.

Considerations:
Sensible precautions apply as with all concentrated essential oils. Refer to Essential Oil Safety Precautions pages 17 and 18.

Cumin -

Cuminum cyminum

Plant Family: Apiaceae (Umbelliferae)

Note   Middle
Odour Intensity   Extremely high

Description:
A delicate annual herb with dark green feathery leaves and pink or white flowers, followed by small narrow seeds. Cumin is native to Egypt, but widely cultivated in the Mediterranean region.

The oil is extracted by steam distillation of the ripe seeds. It is a yellowish green liquid with a warm, spicy-musky aroma reminiscent of Aniseed. Its odour effect is warming and stimulating: a reputed aphrodisiac.

Aromatherapy Uses:
Poor circulation, indigestion, flatulence, headaches, migraine, colds and 'flu, loss of periods outside pregnancy, nervous exhaustion.

Aesthetic Blending Guide:
Cumin blends well with citrus oils, Lavender, Lavandin, Lavender, Ho-leaf, Galbanum, Rosemary, Cardomom, Coriander. The oil is highly odoriferous and will predominate your blends unless used sparingly.

Suggested Massage Oil Blend:
For poor circulation: 25 ml vegetable base oil, 4 drops Cumin, 4 drops Coriander, 5 drops Lavender.

Considerations:
The oil is phototoxic, so do not apply to skin shortly before exposure to natural or simulated sunlight. Avoid during pregnancy.

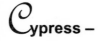ypress –

Cupressus sempervirens

Plant Family: Cupressaceae

Note   Base
Odour Intensity   Medium to low

Nature of Essential the Oil:
Cypress is a tall, evergreen tree with slender branches and a conical shape. It is native to the Mediterranean.

The oil is extracted by steam distillation of the needles, twigs and cones. It is a pale greenish-yellow liquid with a fresh, woody, balsamic aroma. Although the aroma is also somewhat medicinal, it is often described as pleasantly cooling, and calming. Many people perceive it as engendering an expansive sensation.

Aromatherapy Uses:
Skin care (oily skin), acne, poor circulation, excessive perspiration, gum disorders, wounds, bronchitis, spasmodic coughs, rheumatism, excessive menstruation, menopausal distress, nervous tension and other stress-related states. Although the oil is commonly recommended for easing the pain and inflammation of varicose veins and haemorrhoids, it lacks certain water soluble constituents, including tannins, which are regarded as efficacious for these two related ailments. Aqueous extracts of Cypress (as used in herbal medicine) may therefore be more effective.

Aesthetic Blending Guide:
Cypress blends well with Bergamot and other citrus oils, Benzoin, Clary Sage, Frankincense, Petitgrain, Pine, Juniper berry, Lavender, Marjoram, Sandalwood.

Suggested Vaporising Blend:
To facilitate meditation: 3 drops Cypress, 2 drops Frankincense, 2 drops Petitgrain, 3 drops Cedarwood.

Considerations:
Although people who have been exposed to Cypress wood have developed contact dermatitis, The oil is generally regarded as non-irritant and non-sensitising.

ill - *Anethum graveolens*

Plant Family: Apiaceae (Umbelliferae)

Note   Top to middle
Odour Intensity   Medium to high

Description:
Dill is an annual herb, native to the eastern Mediterranean region and western Asia, with furrowed stems, feathery leaves and umbels of yellowish flowers.

The oil is extracted by steam distillation of the fresh or partially dried whole herb or 'weed'. Oil is also distilled from the seed: although for therapeutic purposes, dill weed oil is generally regarded as superior. It is a pale yellow liquid with a sweet-spicy aroma. The odour effect is generally perceived as warming and stimulating.

Aromatherapy Uses:
Fluid retention, bronchitis, indigestion, flatulence, colic, loss of periods outside pregnancy, to promote the flow of breast milk.

Aesthetic Blending Guide
Dill blends well with citrus oils, Basil, Peppermint, sweet Marjoram, Caraway, Nutmeg (and other spices), Lemongrass, Sandalwood.

Suggested Dry Inhalation Blend:
As a supportive remedy to help promote the flow of mother's milk: 2 drops dill, 2 drops Lemongrass. Put the oils on a tissue and inhale at intervals throughout the day.

Considerations:
Sensible precautions apply as with all concentrated essential oils. Refer to Essential Oil Safety Precautions pages 17 and 18.

$\mathscr{E}$ucalyptus, Blue Gum -

Eucalyptus globulus

Plant Family: Myrtaceae

Note   Top
Odour Intensity   High

Nature of Essential the Oil:
A tall evergreen tree with bluish-green, sword-shaped leaves and creamy white flowers. The tree is native to Australia and Tasmania and is also cultivated in Africa, Spain, Portugal, Brazil, California and China, from where much of the world's supply of eucalyptus oil is produced.

The oil is extracted by steam distillation of the leaves and young twigs. It is a virtually colourless liquid. The aroma is piercing and camphoraceous with a woody undertone. Its odour effect is head-clearing and cooling.

Aromatherapy Uses:
Burns, blisters, chickenpox, measles, cold sores, cuts, insect bites and stings, insect repellent, headlice, skin infections, wounds, arthritic pain, muscular aches and pains, sprains, poor circulation, cystitis, hay fever, colds and 'flu, headaches, neuralgia, as a fumigant when infectious illness is around.

Aesthetic Blending Guide:
This variety of Eucalyptus blends well with Cedarwood, Frankincense, Lavender, Lemon, Marjoram, Myrrh, Pine, Rosemary, Thyme.

Suggested Massage Oil/Vaporising Blend:
A chest rub for cold and 'flu symptoms, acute bronchitis and catarrh: 25 ml vegetable base oil, 5 drops Eucalyptus, 4 drops Myrrh, 3 drops Lavender. This same combination can be used in the vaporiser to ease breathing and fumigate the air.

Considerations:
Eucalyptus oil is generally regarded as non-irritant and non-sensitising. However, it must never be taken internally as relatively tiny amounts can be fatal, especially to children. Anecdotal evidence suggests that the oil can irritate skin if used in the bath.

$\mathcal{E}$ucalyptus, Lemon-Scented -   *Eucalyptus citriodora*

Plant Family: Myrtaceae

Note   Top
Odour Intensity   High

Description:
A tall evergreen tree with an impressively straight trunk. The young leaves are oval, the mature leaves narrow and tapering. Lemon-scented eucalyptus is native to Australia, though cultivated mainly in Brazil and China.

The oil is extracted by steam distillation of the leaves and twigs. It is a colourless to pale yellow liquid with a strong, Citronella-like aroma. Its odour effect is head-clearing and refreshing.

Aromatherapy Uses:
Athlete's foot, cuts and grazes, arthritic pain, muscular aches and pains, bronchitis, coughs, throat infections, colds and 'flu, headaches, insect repellent, as a fumigant when infectious illness is around.

Aesthetic Blending Guide:
This variety of Eucalyptus has a powerful aroma and therefore does not blend very well with other essences. However, it is acceptable when carefully blended with Geranium, Palmarosa, Cedarwood, Cypress, Pine or Tea Tree.

Suggested Vaporising Blend:
As a fumigant when infectious illness is around (e.g. measles, colds and 'flu): 5 drops Eucalyptus citriodora, 5 drops Tea Tree, 5 drops Pine.

Considerations:
Skin applications of the oil may cause sensitisation reactions. Do not use in the bath as it may irritate the skin. Eucalyptus oil can be highly toxic when taken internally (see Eucalyptus globulus).

$\mathcal{F}$ennel, Sweet -

Plant Family: Apiaceae (Umbelliferar)

Note   Middle
Odour Intensity   High

Description:
A tall perennial herb with feathery leaves and umbels of yellowish flowers. The small brown seeds are curved and ribbed.

The essential oil is captured by steam distillation of the crushed seeds. It is a virtually colourless liquid with a pungent aroma reminiscent of Aniseed, but with a camphor-like undertone. The odour effect is warming and stimulating.

Aromatherapy Uses:
As a supportive remedy for detoxification purposes, fluid retention, bruises, gum disease, offensive breath, rheumatism, bronchitis, to promote appetite after illness, colic, flatulence, loss of periods outside pregnancy, to promote the flow of breast milk (but see Considerations).

Aesthetic Blending Guide:
Fennel does not blend well with many oils because of its distinctive and overpowering aroma. However, it is acceptable if used sparingly with Lavender, Geranium or Sandalwood.

Suggested Mouthwash Blend:
To help treat gingivitis: Put 1 teaspoon of cider vinegar into a teacup. Add 1 drop of Fennel and 1 drop of Geranium and stir well. Top up with warm water and use as a mouthwash. Swish around your mouth, and then spit it out. Repeat several times, or until the mixture is used up. Use the mouthwash two or three times a day, making a fresh batch each time.

Considerations:
The oil may irritate sensitive skin. Never use in the bath as it tends to cause a stinging sensation, triggered by the heat and humidity. There is a remote possibility that Fennel may trigger an epileptic seizure in those prone to the condition. For skin applications, use in the lowest recommended concentrations of around 0.5% (i.e. 1 drop in 2 or 3 teaspoons of carrier oil). When using the oil to help increase the flow of breast milk, it is advisable to avoid skin applications. Instead, put a few drops on a handkerchief and inhale at intervals throughout the day. Avoid during pregnancy.

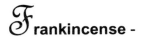# $\mathscr{F}$rankincense -

Boswellia carterii

Synonyms:

Olibanum
(only from Somalia),
Encens, Incense.

Plant Family:

Burseraceae

Note   Base
Odour Intensity   High

Description:
The oil is extracted by steam distillation of frankincense 'tears' - little pieces of solidified oleo gum resin which exude from natural fissures in the bark of the small tree. Frankincense is native to the arid regions of Arabia and North Africa. The oil is a colourless to pale yellow liquid with a warm, balsamic, camphoraceous aroma. Unlike most other essential oils, the aroma of Frankincense improves with age. Its odour effect is warming, head-clearing and calming.

Aromatherapy Uses:
Skin care (particularly mature skin), acne, abscesses, scars, wounds, haemorrhoids, respiratory ailments such as asthma, bronchitis, coughs, catarrh and laryngitis, cystitis, painful menstruation, spotting in between periods, pre-menstrual syndrome, nervous tension and other stress-related states. A popular Vaporising oil with an ancient reputation for aiding meditation From this author's experience, Frankincense also makes an excellent massage oil for easing arthritic and rheumatic pain.

Aesthetic Blending Guide:
Frankincense blends well with Benzoin, citrus oils, Coriander and other spice oils, Basil, Cedarwood, Cypress, Galbanum, Geranium, Juniper, Lavender, Neroli, Palmarosa, Patchouli, Petitgrain Rose, Sandalwood, Vetiver.

Suggested Massage Oil Blend:
To help engender deep relaxation: 25ml vegetable base oil, 3 drops Frankincense, 3 drops Neroli (or Petitgrain), 3 drops Mandarin.

Considerations:
Avoid skin applications during the first trimester of pregnancy.

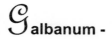**albanum -**   *Ferula galbaniflua*

Plant Family: Apiaceae (Umbelliferae)

Note   Base
Odour Intensity   Extremely high

Description:
A large perennial herb with umbels of small white flowers. Galbanum is native to the Middle East and western Asia.

The oil is extracted by steam distillation of the oleoresin (a gum which is collected after incisions are made in the thick stalks of the plant). It is an olive green, slightly viscous liquid. Its aroma is very powerful, reminiscent of dense green undergrowth with a dry earthy quality. The odour effect is head-clearing, and yet also very calming and grounding.

Aromatherapy Uses:
Skin care (especially mature skin), abscesses, acne, boils, to encourage the formation of scar tissue (an essential process in the healing of wounds), cuts and sores, inflamed skin, skin ulcers, insect stings and bites, poor circulation, muscular aches and pains, rheumatism, respiratory ailments, indigestion, flatulence, bronchitis, catarrh, chronic coughs, loss of periods outside of pregnancy, nervous tension and other stress-related states. It can also be used in a vaporiser to facilitate meditation.

Aesthetic Blending Guide:
Galbanum blends well with Bergamot (and other citrus oils), Cedarwood, Clary Sage, Cypress, Lavender, Frankincense, Petitgrain, Pine, Geranium. However, the oil is exceptionally odoriferous and will overpower your blends unless used in minute quantities. For instance, as little as 1 drop in 25-30 ml of carrier oil, blended with other oils.

Suggested Massage Oil Blend:
A deeply relaxing blend: 25 ml vegetable base oil, 1 drop Galbanum, 3 drops Frankincense, 3 drops Petitgrain, 3 drops Lavender.

Considerations:
The oil is generally regarded as non-irritant and non-sensitising. However, since Galbanum reputedly stimulates menstruation, it is advisable to avoid during pregnancy.

$\mathcal{G}$eranium -

Pelargonium graveolens

Synonyms: Bourbon Geranium,
                                                 Rose Geranium.

Plant Family: Geraniaceae

Other Species:
There are a number of oil-producing pelargoniums,
including *P. odorantissimum*, *P. Roseum*, *P. radens*, and various hybrid varieties.

Note   Middle to top
Odour Intensity   High

Description:
A spreading shrub with pointed leaves, serrated at the edges, and small rose-pink flowers. The plant is native to South Africa.

The oil is extracted by steam distillation of the leaves, stalks and flowers. It is a greenish-olive liquid with a piercingly sweet and rosy scent. Bourbon Geranium, which is generally regarded as having the best quality of aroma, also emits a background nuance of mint. Geranium's odour effect is refreshing and uplifting. Intriguingly, it can be relaxing to some people and enlivening to others.

Aromatherapy Uses:
Skin care (most skin types), burns, headlice, ringworm, neuralgia, poor circulation, engorgement of the breasts, menopausal distress, pre-menstrual syndrome, nervous tension, mild depression and other stress-related states.

Aesthetic Blending Guide:
Geranium blends well with many essences, but especially Coriander, citrus essences, Neroli, Patchouli, Petitgrain, Rosemary, Sandalwood, Vetiver, Ylang Ylang.

Suggested Massage Oil/Dry Inhalation Blend:
An enlivening, sunny formula helpful for mild depression, especially the 'winter blues': 25 ml vegetable base oil, 3 drops Geranium, 2 drops Neroli (or Petitgrain), 3 drops Sweet Orange, 1 drop Rosemary. Alternatively, put the same combination of undiluted essential oils on to a handkerchief and inhale at intervals throughout the day.

Considerations:
The oil is highly odoriferous and may irritate sensitive skin. Always use in the lowest recommended concentrations.

$\mathcal{G}$inger -

Plant Family: Zingiberaceae

Note   Middle to base
Odour Intensity   Very high

Description:
A tall reed-like plant, stemming from tuberous rhizomes. Ginger is native to southern Asia, though it is also cultivated commercially in the West Indies and Africa.

The oil is extracted by steam distillation of the dried, ground rhizomes. It is a pale amber liquid with a pungent, warm and spicy aroma. However, it lacks the fruity odour nuance found in the raw plant material because the process of distillation alters its original chemical structure. The odour effect is warming and stimulating: a reputed aphrodisiac.

Aromatherapy Uses:
Arthritic and rheumatic pain, muscular aches and pains, poor circulation, catarrh, coughs, sore throat, diarrhoea, colic, indigestion, loss of appetite, nausea, travel sickness, colds and 'flu, mental fatigue, nervous exhaustion. It can also be vaporised as a fumigant when infectious illness is around.

Aesthetic Blending Guide:
Ginger blends well with Cedarwood, Coriander and other spices, Cinnamon, citrus essences, Frankincense, Neroli, Patchouli, Petitgrain, Rose, Sandalwood, Vetiver, Ylang Ylang. The oil is highly odoriferous, so use sparingly.

Suggested Aromatic Bath:
For helping to alleviate cold or 'flu symptoms: 1 drop Ginger, 1 drop Cardomom, 3 drops Coriander, 3 drops Sweet Orange.

Considerations:
The oil may irritate sensitive skin. Use in the lowest recommended concentrations. The oil is mildly phototoxic, but only if applied to skin neat or in high concentrations.

$\mathcal{G}$rapefruit -

Citrus x paradisi

Plant Family: Rutaceae

Note   Top
Odour Intensity Medium

Description:
A hybrid citrus tree, thought to be a cross between *C. grandis* and *C. sinensis*. It has glossy leaves, fragrant white flowers and large yellow fruits. The vast majority of the oil is produced in Florida and Israel.

The oil is extracted by cold expression of the fresh peel of the fruit. It is a pale yellow or greenish liquid with a fresh, sweet and citrus fragrance. Its odour effect is uplifting and refreshing. An inferior grade essential oil can be steam distilled from the fruit pulp, which contains oil bearing peel fragments.

Aromatherapy Uses:
Colds and 'flu, mild depression, nervous exhaustion. Reputedly helpful for cellulite, but in this author's experience professional lymphatic drainage massage (with or without essential oils) is far more effective.

Aesthetic Blending Guide:
Grapefruit blends well with other citrus essences, Cardomom, Coriander, Cypress, Juniper, Lavender, Neroli, Petitigrain, Pine, Geranium, Rosemary, Tea Tree.

Suggested Vaporising Blend:
A cooling and enlivening room scent: 5 drops Grapefruit, 1 drop Lime, 3 drops Scots Pine

Considerations:
Expressed oil of Grapefruit is slightly phototoxic and must not be applied to skin shortly before exposure to natural or simulated sunlight as it may promote unsightly pigmentation. The distilled oil, however, is non-phototoxic. Grapefruit oil, like most other citrus essences (excepting Bergamot), has a relatively short shelf-life and must be used up within 6-9 months of purchase. Once oxidised, it is much more likely to irritate the skin.

69

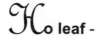 **o leaf -** *Cinnamomum camphora var. galvescens*

Plant Family: Lauraceae

Note — Middle to top
Odour Intensity — Medium

Description:
The oil is extracted by steam distillation of the leaves of a tall, evergreen tree native to the Far East. It is a pale yellow liquid with a sweet woody-floral fragrance. Its odour effect is generally described as uplifting and enlivening.

NB Aromatherapists are increasingly turning to this oil as a sustainable alternative to the essential oil of Rosewood (*Aniba rosaeodora*), which is obtained from threatened species found growing in the rainforests of South America. Both oils have a similar chemical composition.

Aromatherapy Uses:
Ho leaf oil is said to be a tissue regenerator, and thus it is often used in cosmetic formulations for mature skin. Also helpful for feverish ailments such as colds and 'flu, mild depression, anxiety and nervous tension.

Aesthetic Blending Guide:
Ho leaf oil blends especially well with Bergamot (and other citrus oils), Sandalwood, Cedarwood, Pine, Rose, Jasmine, Neroli, Frankincense, Geranium, Lavender.

Suggested Massage Oil Blend:
A face and neck formulation for mature skin: 25 ml vegetable base oil (e.g. Rosehip, Sweet Almond, Apricot), 3 drops Ho leaf, 1 drop Rose Otto, 1 drop Sandalwood, 1 drop Frankincense.

Considerations:
There is no traditional therapeutic use of Ho leaf oil (or Rosewood), as both oils are primarily regarded as perfumery materials. The therapeutic information given here derives from anecdotal evidence. However, perfume chemists generally regard the oil as non-toxic, non-irritant and non-sensitising.

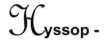yssop -

Hyssopus officinalis

Plant Family: Lamiaceae (Labiatae)

Note   Middle
Odour Intensity   High

Description:
A perennial woody herb with small lance-shaped leaves and purplish-blue flowers. Hyssop is native to the Mediterranean region and temperate Asia.

The oil is extracted by steam distillation of the leaves and flowering tops. It is a colourless to pale yellow liquid with a sweet, camphoraceous top note and spicy undertone. Its odour effect is warming and restorative.

Aromatherapy Uses:
Bruises, cuts, wounds, low or high blood pressure (it has a stabilising effect), rheumatic aches and pains, bronchitis, asthma (but only under strict professional supervision), catarrh, coughs, sore throat, tonsillitis, whooping cough, indigestion, delayed menstruation outside pregnancy, colds and 'flu, nervous exhaustion and other stress-related states.

Aesthetic Blending Guide:
Hyssop blends well with Clary Sage, Bay, Bergamot, Lemon, Grapefruit, Geranium, Lavender, myrtle, Rosemary.

Suggested Vaporising Blend:
A fumigant to vaporise when infectious illness is around, or simply as a refreshing room scent: 3 drops Hyssop, 3 drops Lemon, 2 drops Rosemary.

Considerations:
Hyssop essential oil is quite toxic and is therefore usually sold as a 'restricted' product, reserved solely for professional use. However, it is safe if used in moderation (i.e. a few drops blended with other compatible oils) in a purpose designed essential oil vaporiser. Nevertheless, it's best avoided altogether during pregnancy. The oil reputedly provokes seizures in predisposed individuals, so must be avoided by epileptics.

nula -   *Inula graveolens* or *I. odorata*

Plant Family: Asteraceae (Compositae)

Note   Middle
Odour Intensity   High

Description:
A perennial herb with a stout stem and large, yellow, daisy-like flowers. The plant is native to Europe and Asia.

The oil is extracted by steam distillation of the dried roots and rhizomes. It is a bluish green liquid with a gentle woody, honey-like aroma. Its odour effect is soothing and cooling.

Aromatherapy Uses:
Catarrh, coughs, colds, sinusitis, earache, bronchitis, feverish ailments (including 'flu), high blood pressure, nervous tension and anxiety.

Aesthetic Blending Guide:
Inula blends well with Bergamot, Cedarwood, Cinnamon, Ciste, Clary Sage, Coriander, Cypress, Sandalwood, Patchouli, Lavender, Frankincense, Ylang Ylang.

Suggested Steam Inhalation Blend:
Especially helpful for spasmodic coughs (including whooping cough), 'flu, bronchitis and sinusitis: 2 drops Inula, 1 drop Cypress, 1 drop Lavender.

Considerations:
Often sold as a 'restricted' oil, solely for professional use. This is because it is closely related to Elecampane (I.helenium), which is known to be a severe skin sensitiser. However, the variety of Inula profiled here is generally regarded as safe, at least when used in steam inhalations or as a Vaporising oil. Nevertheless, being a newcomer to aromatherapy, it is advisable to err on the side of caution and avoid using the oil in such applications as massage blends, baths and ointments.

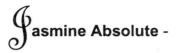 asmine Absolute -

Jasminum officinale

Plant Family: Oleaceae

Note   Base to middle
Odour Intensity   High

Description:
An evergreen climber which produces an abundance of white star-shaped flowers whose rich fragrance intensifies after dusk. Jasmine is native to China, northern India and the Middle East.

The Absolute is captured by solvent extraction of the flowers. It is an Orangey-brown, viscous liquid. The tenacious fragrance is richly floral with a pronounced musky note. Its odour effect is warming and intoxicating: a reputed aphrodisiac.

Aromatherapy Uses:
Although believed to be helpful for muscular aches and pains, catarrh, coughs and laryngitis, there are many other less expensive oils which can be used for such ailments. Jasmine absolute also has a reputation for facilitating childbirth. In the traditional medicine of India, Jasmine flowers are applied as a compress to arrest the flow of breast milk, which suggests that the absolute possibly exerts the same effect. Certainly, Jasmine reigns supreme as a mood-elevating aromatic for such conditions as mild depression, pre-menstrual syndrome and stress-related states.

Aesthetic Blending Guide:
Jasmine blends well with other floral essences, citrus essences, Black Pepper, Clary Sage and Sandalwood.

Suggested Vaporising Blend:
A voluptuous aphrodisiac blend: 3 drops Jasmine absolute, 3 drops Rose absolute (or 1-2 drops Rose Otto), 3 drops Sandalwood. This blend is even more sensational if vaporised in a 50/50 mix of Rosewater and Orange flower water instead of the usual tap water.

Considerations:
Avoid skin applications during pregnancy and while breast feeding. This method should also be avoided by those with sensitive skin. Unfortunately, because of the high price of Jasmine absolute, it is especially vulnerable to adulteration.

$\int$uniper -

Juniperus communis

Plant Family: Cupressaceae

Note   Base to middle
Odour Intensity   Medium to high

Description:
A small evergreen conifer tree, with bluish-green needles and bluish-black berries. Juniper is native to North America, Europe (including Britain), northern Asia, Korea and Japan.

The highest grade of **Juniper Berry** oil is extracted by steam distillation of the crushed, dried (or partially dried) fruits. An inferior oil is captured by steam distillation of the fermented berries (as a by-product of gin manufacture).
An oil is also extracted from the needles and wood and labelled **'Juniper Needle'**. Juniper berry and Juniper needle oils are virtually colourless. Top grade Juniper berry oil has the finest aroma. It is fresh and woody with a pleasant Peppery overtone. Its odour effect is uplifting, and yet also warming and calming: a reputed aphrodisiac. The less expensive Juniper needle has a comparatively harsh, turpentine-like aroma. Its odour effect is invigorating.

Aromatherapy Uses:
Although the oils of Juniper berry and Juniper needle have similar therapeutic properties, most aromatherapists favour the former. It is used for skin and hair care (oily), acne, weeping eczema, haemorrhoids, wounds, cellulite, arthritic and rheumatic complaints, muscular aches and pains, loss of periods outside pregnancy, painful menstruation, cystitis, pre-menstrual syndrome, nervous tension and other stress-related states.

Aesthetic Blending Guide:
Juniper needle has a much stronger aroma and needs to be used in tiny quantities, otherwise it will predominate your blends. Both Juniper needle and Juniper berry oils blend well with Benzoin, citrus oils, Cedarwood, Cypress, Frankincense, Geranium, Lavender, Neroli, Petitgrain, Pine, Rosemary, Sandalwood, Vetiver.

Suggested Massage Oil Blend:
For reducing stress levels and uplifting the spirits: 25 ml vegetable base oil, 3 drops Juniper berry oil, 4 drops Bergamot FCF, 2 drops Neroli.

Considerations:
Avoid skin applications during pregnancy as the oil may stimulate the uterus. This method should also be avoided by those with kidney disease: there is a chance that it may exacerbate the condition if used without specialist knowledge. It is essential to buy essential oil of Juniper from a reputable supplier. For although it is often cited as being irritant to skin, this may be due to the fact it is commonly adulterated with turpentine.

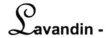**avandin -** *Lavandula angustifolia* x *L. latifolia*

Plant Family: Lamiaceae (Labiatae)

Note   Middle
Odour Intensity Medium to High

Description:
The oil is extracted by steam distillation of the fresh flowering tops of a hybrid Lavender (a cross between True and Spike Lavenders). It gives a higher yield of oil than either true Lavender (*L. angustifolia*) or spike Lavender (*L. latifolia*). The oil is colourless to pale yellow with a fresh, camphoraceous top note, and a woody undertone. Although not as popular as true Lavender, whose fragrance is sweeter, the odour effect of Lavandin is generally perceived as uplifting and refreshing.

Aromatherapy Uses:
Lavandin has been around for less than 70 years, so does not have a long history of use.   Although it shares many of the properties of true Lavender, most aromatherapists prefer to use it solely as a Vaporising oil - to purify the air and repel insects.   However, it is also helpful for muscular aches and pains, minor burns, bruises, nervous tension and other stress-related states.

Aesthetic Blending Guide:
Lavandin blends well with Bergamot, Lime, Lemon, Clary Sage, Clove, Bay, Cinnamon, Coriander, Citronella, Lemongrass, Palmarosa, Cypress, Pine, Thyme, Rosemary.
Suggested Vaporising Blend: To repel insects: 4 drops Lavandin, 2 drops Lemongrass, 2 drops Palmarosa.

Considerations:
Unfortunately, the less expensive Lavandin is sometimes sold at an inflated price in the name of true Lavender, L. angustifolia. But to the experienced nose, the oils are distinctly different. To better enable detection of a mislabelled product, it is advisable to become familiar with the aromas of both types of Lavender oil.

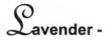 **avender -** *Lavandula angustifolia*

Plant Family: Lamiaceae (Labiatae)

Note   Middle
Odour Intensity   Medium to high

Description:
An evergreen, woody shrub producing abundant spikes of bluish-mauve flowers. Lavender is native to the Mediterranean.

The oil is extracted by steam distillation of the flowering tops. It is a pale yellow liquid with a sweet floral-herbaceous fragrance. Its odour effect is uplifting, calming and refreshing.

Aromatherapy Uses:
Skin care (most skin types), acne, allergies, athlete's foot, boils, bruises, eczema, dandruff, burns, chilblains ringworm, scabies, insect bites and stings, as an insect repellent, asthma, earache, coughs, colds and 'flu, catarrh, laryngitis, muscular aches and pains, rheumatic pain, nausea, colic, cystitis, painful menstruation, mild depression, headache, insomnia, migraine, pre-menstrual syndrome, nervous tension and other stress-related states.

Aesthetic Blending Guide:
Lavender blends with most other essences, especially Cedarwood, Chamomile (Roman and German), Clary Sage, Clove bud, Coriander, Cypress, Frankincense, Geranium, Juniper, Mimosa, Neroli, Rose, Petitgrain, Pine, Vetiver.

Suggested Massage Oil Blend:
For muscular aches and pains and to soothe nervous tension: 25 ml vegetable base oil, 5 drops Lavender, 2 drops Frankincense, 2 drops Clary Sage.

Considerations:
Generally regarded as non-irritant and non-sensitising. However, there are reports of contact dermatitis as a result of over-use of the oil, especially amongst aromatherapists themselves. It is also possible to be sensitive to one particular brand of Lavender and not to another, even though both types may be labelled *'L. officinalis'*. This may suggest that the oil has been adulterated or that it has oxidised. The oil is much more likely to irritate skin when used neat or in high concentrations.

Lemon -

Plant Family: Rutaceae

Note   Top
Odour Intensity   Medium to high

Description:
A small evergreen tree producing fragrant white flowers, followed by the yellow fruit. Lemon is native to Asia, but has become naturalised in the Mediterranean region. It is predominantly produced in California, South Africa and the Ivory Coast.

The preferred expressed oil is extracted by cold expression of the fresh peel of the fruit. It is a pale yellow liquid with a fresh, sharp aroma just like the freshly grated zest. Its odour effect is uplifting and cooling. An inferior grade essential oil can be steam distilled from the fruit pulp, which contains oil bearing peel fragments.

Aromatherapy Uses:
Skin care (oily skin), acne, boils, chilblains, cellulite, arthritis, high blood pressure, poor circulation, rheumatic and arthritic aches and pains, sore throat, bronchitis, catarrh, colds and 'flu, nervous tension, mild depression.

Aesthetic Blending Guide:
Lemon blends well with other citrus essences, Roman Chamomile, Cypress, Frankincense, Juniper, Lavender, Myrrh, Neroli, Petitgrain, Pine, Rose, Sage, Sandalwood, Tea Tree, Ylang Ylang.

Suggested Vaporising Blend:
To soothe nervous tension and anxiety: 5 drops Lemon, 2 drops Sandalwood, 3 drops Ylang Ylang.

Considerations:
Like most other expressed citrus oils, Lemon essence is phototoxic. Do not apply to skin shortly before exposure to natural or simulated sunlight as it may cause unsightly pigmentation. The distilled oil is non-phototoxic. Lemon oil has a short shelf-life and should be used up within 6-9 months of purchase. Once oxidised, it is much more likely to irritate the skin. For skin applications, always use in the lowest recommended concentrations.

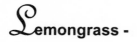 **emongrass -** *Cymbopogon flexuosus*

Plant Family: Poaceae (Gramineae)

Note   Top to middle
Odour Intensity   Very high

Description:
A fast growing aromatic grass native to tropical Asia, though cultivated in other areas. Most of the oil, whether 'West Indian' or 'East Indian' is produced in Guatemala and India.

The oil is extracted by steam distillation of the fresh and partially dried grass, finely chopped. It is a yellow or light amber liquid. The aroma is sweet and Lemony with a grassy undertone. Its odour effect is uplifting and refreshing, albeit less so than pure Lemon oil. Some people find the aroma quite relaxing, other regard it as enlivening.

Aromatherapy Uses:
Athlete's foot, insect repellent, scabies, muscular aches and pains, poor circulation, insufficient milk in breastfeeding mothers, indigestion, fevers, as a fumigant when infectious illness is around, headaches, nervous exhaustion and other stress-related states.

Aesthetic Blending Guide:
It blends well with Bergamot and other citrus essences, Cardomom, Chamomile (Roman and German), Clove, Coriander, Eucalyptus, Geranium, Ginger, Lavender, Myrrh, Palmarosa, Patchouli, Petitgrain, Rosemary. The aroma is highly odoriferous and will predominate your blends unless used sparingly.

Suggested Massage Oil Blend:
For overworked muscles and/or nervous exhaustion: 25 ml vegetable base oil, 2 drops Lemongrass, 5 drops Mandarin, 2 drops Rosemary.

Considerations:
The oil may irritate sensitive skin. Use in the lowest recommended concentrations. The potential irritant effect of the oil is lessened if blended with an equal quantity (at least) of Mandarin essence.

ime -

Citrus aurantifolia

Plant Family: Rutaceae

Note   Top
Odour Intensity   High

Description:
A small evergreen citrus tree with glossy leaves, fragrant white flowers and green fruit. The tree is native to Asia. The main production area is Mexico, then Haiti. The West Indies and Peru also produce Lime oil, but to a much lesser degree.

There are two methods of extraction: cold expression and steam distillation. Both oils are extracted from the fresh peel of the fruit. Although the expressed oil has a superior aroma, the distilled essence is much safer for use on the skin (see Considerations). The distilled oil is virtually colourless whereas the expressed essence is Olive green. The odour effect (of both grades) is uplifting and refreshing.

Aromatherapy Uses:
Colds and 'flu, poor circulation, high blood pressure, mild depression, nervous exhaustion and other stress-related states.

Aesthetic Blending Guide:
Lime oil blends well with other citrus essences, Neroli, Geranium, Petitgrain, Lavender, Rosemary, Clary Sage, Ylang Ylang.

Suggested Vaporising Blend:
A sweet and refreshing room scent ideal for summer days: 4 drops Lime, 1 drop Neroli, 2 drops Geranium, 2 drops Ylang Ylang.

Considerations:
The expressed oil is highly phototoxic and must never be applied to skin shortly before exposure to natural or simulated sunlight. However, the distilled oil is non-phototoxic. Both types are potentially irritant to skin, so use in low concentrations. The expressed oil has a very short shelf-life and must be used up within six months. The distilled essence will keep for up to one year.

$\mathcal{L}$ime Blossom (Linden) Absolute -

Tilia cordata

Plant Family: Tiliaceae

Note   Base to middle
Odour Intensity   High

Description:
The lime (also known as linden) is a tall woodland tree, producing an abundance of fragrant, creamy white flowers. It is native to Europe, Siberia and Asia.

The Absolute is produced by solvent extraction of the dried. Not to be confused with *Citrus aurantifolia*, the tree which produces the fruit we call Limes. Lime blossom absolute is a yellow, viscous substance with a sweet, hay-like fragrance. Its odour effect is soothing and intoxicating.

Aromatherapy Uses:
Not much used in aromatherapy, mainly because of its high price and because it is especially vulnerable to adulteration. Reputedly helpful for insomnia, nervous tension and other stress-related states.

Aesthetic blending Guide:
Lime blossom absolute is a wonderful ingredient for creating mood-enhancing room fragrances. It blends well with other floral absolutes, also with citrus essences, Cedarwood, Geranium, Sandalwood, Ylang Ylang.

Suggested Vaporising Blend:
A luxuriously sweet blend to lull you into a quiet reverie: 2 drops Linden absolute, 1 drop Ylang Ylang, 2 drops Sandalwood, 4 drops Mandarin.

Considerations:
Unfortunately there is no safety data available at present. It may therefore be advisable to avoid skin applications of the absolute and to use it solely as a Vaporising aromatic. Otherwise, use in very low concentrations of around 0.5% (i.e.1 drop per 10 ml base oil), or even less.

$\mathcal{L}$itsea cubeba -

Litsea cubeba

Synonym: Mai Chang

Plant Family: Lauraceae

Note   Middle to top
Odour Intensity   High

Description:
A small tropical tree with fragrant lemongrass-scented leaves and flowers. The flowers are followed by small fruits shaped like peppers. Litsea cubeba is native to Asia, especially China.

The oil is extracted by steam distillation of the leaves and flowers. It is a pale yellow liquid with an intensely sweet fragrance reminiscent of Lemongrass. The odour effect is uplifting and cooling.

Aromatherapy Uses:
Excessively oily skin, flatulence, indigestion, as an insect repellent, and as a fumigant when infectious illness is around.

Aesthetic Blending Guide:
Litsea cubeba blends well with Bergamot, Benzoin, Cedarwood, Frankincense, Orange, Tea Tree, Geranium, Mandarin or Petitgrain.

Suggested Vaporising Blend:
A fresh-smelling blend which can be vaporised as a fumigant when infectious illness is around: 4 drops Litsea cubeba, 3 drops Tea Tree, 2 drops Petitgrain, 4 drops Bergamot.

Considerations:
For skin applications, use in the lowest recommended concentrations. The oil is best avoided by those with sensitive skin or eczema.

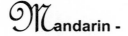andarin -

Citrus reticulata

Plant Family: Rutaceae

Note   Top
Odour Intensity   Very low

Description:
A small evergreen tree with glossy leaves and fragrant white flowers, followed by the fleshy fruit. Native to China, though now cultivated mainly in the Mediterranean.

The oil is extracted by cold expression of the rind of the fruit. It can be a green, orange or yellow liquid with a gentle, sweet citrus scent. Its odour effect is soothing and uplifting.

Aromatherapy Uses:
Oily skin conditions, prevention of stretch marks during pregnancy, indigestion, insomnia, nervous tension.

Aesthetic Blending Guide:
Mandarin blends well with other citrus oils, also Lavender, Petitgrain and Neroli. However, the aroma is of very low intensity and therefore benefits from being blended with more tenacious essences such as Basil, Cedarwood, Black Pepper, Coriander, Frankincense, Rose Otto, Rose absolute, Rosemary, Sandalwood, Lemongrass, Palmarosa, Ylang Ylang

Suggested Massage Oil Blend:
A deeply relaxing formula with sensuous notes: 25 ml vegetable base oil, 5 drops Mandarin, 2 drops Sandalwood, 2 drops Cedarwood, 1 drop Rose Otto (or 2 drops Rose absolute).

Considerations:
The oil is slightly phototoxic and may cause unsightly pigmentation if applied to skin shortly before exposure to natural or simulated sunlight. Like most other citrus essences, it has a relatively short shelf-life, especially once the bottle has been opened and the contents exposed to air. Therefore, it is best used up within 8 months of purchase.

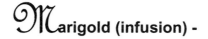arigold (infusion) - *Calendula officinalis*

Plant Family: Asteraceae (Compositae)

Other Names for the Product:
Marigold (or Calendula) maceration, marigold (or Calendula) macerated oil.

Description:
Calendula is an annual herb with pale green leaves and bright orange or yellow daisy-like flowers. Although native to southern Europe the plant is now grown in gardens everywhere.

Nature of the Aromatic Oil:
The oil is prepared by macerating the flower heads in a vegetable base oil (usually Sunflower or Olive) until the properties of the plant material are imparted to the oil, after which time the product is filtered and bottled. The oil is golden yellow with a dry, honey-like aroma.

Aromatherapy Uses:
To soothe and heal sore, inflamed and itchy skin conditions, such as eczema, nappy rash, athlete's foot (the oil has anti-fungal properties), sore and cracked nipples (when breastfeeding), and to treat insect bites, minor burns and bruises. It can also be massaged into the hands after heavy outdoor work when there may be little cuts and abrasions. A traditional treatment for varicose veins (reduces inflammation) and for strengthening fragile capillaries on skin prone to thread veins.

Aesthetic Blending Guide:
The aroma and properties of marigold infusion can be enhanced with the addition of a tiny amount   of any of the following oils: Chamomile (Roman or German), Helichrysum, Lavender, Rose Otto.

Suggested Body Oil Blend:
Generally, you will need no more than 1 drop of essential oil per 15-20 ml of marigold infusion. For example, to reinforce the oil's anti-inflammatory properties, add 1 drop of German Chamomile essential oil to every 20 ml of Calendula infusion.

Considerations:
Essential oil of marigold is unavailable because the heat of steam distillation destroys many of the plant's properties. However, a tiny amount of solvent-extracted marigold absolute is produced each year for the perfume industry, although this is rarely available to aromatherapy suppliers. Not to be confused with Tagetes (*Tagetes minuta*), the Mexican marigold, which is a potentially toxic essential oil.

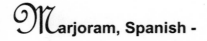arjoram, Spanish -

Thymus mastichina

Plant Family: Lamiaceae (Labiatae)

Note   Top
Odour Intensity   High

Description:
A perennial, bushy herb with small, narrow leaves and numerous little mauve flowers. The plant is native to the Mediterranean.

The oil is extracted by steam distillation of the leaves and flowering tops. It is a pale yellow liquid turning darker with age. The aroma is dry and camphoraceous. Its odour effect is penetrating and head-clearing.

Aromatherapy Uses:
Arthritic and rheumatic pain, muscular aches and pains, poor circulation, bronchitis, catarrh, coughs, colds and 'flu, infectious illness, nervous exhaustion. Reputedly, the oil promotes delayed menstruation.

Aesthetic Blending Guide:
Spanish Marjoram has a rather medicinal aroma which can be improved by blending with larger quantities of oils such as Bergamot, Lavandin, Lavender or Lemon. It also blends quite well with Cedarwood, Pine, Rosemary and Tea Tree.

Suggested Vaporising Blend:
A decongestive, disinfectant formula to vaporise as a fumigant when infectious illness is around. 4 drops Spanish Marjoram, 4 drops Lemon, 3 drops Tea Tree, 4 drops Pine.

Considerations:
As its botanical name confirms, the common name of this plant is a misnomer. It is actually a variety of Thyme and must therefore be regarded with a degree of caution. Unfortunately, its chemistry is unpredictable and can vary from one harvest to another. For example, some batches of Spanish Marjoram oil contain high concentrations of cineole, a substance which is believed to account for its potentially irritant effect on the skin. Use well diluted for local applications, or use solely as a Vaporising oil. Best avoided during pregnancy.

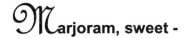arjoram, sweet -   *Origanum majorana*

Plant Family: Lamiaceae (Labiatae)

Note   Top to middle
Odour Intensity   Medium to high

Description:
A tender bushy herb with dark green oval leaves and small greyish-white flowers produced in clusters or 'knots'. The plant is native to the Mediterranean.

The oil is extracted by steam distillation of the dried flowering herb. It is a light amber liquid with a warm, woody and camphoraceous aroma. Its odour effect is warming and calming. It is a reputed anaphrodisiac (quelling sexual desire).

Aromatherapy Uses:
Chilblains, bruises, arthritic and rheumatic pain, muscular aches and pains, sprains and strains, bronchitis, coughs, colic, constipation, flatulence, absence of periods outside pregnancy, painful menstruation, pre-menstrual syndrome, colds and 'flu, headache, high blood pressure, insomnia, migraine, nervous tension and other stress-related states.

Aesthetic Blending Guide:
Sweet Marjoram blends well with Bergamot, Cedarwood, Cypress, Chamomile (Roman and German), Eucalyptus, Juniper (berry and needle), Lavender, Rosemary, Tea Tree.

Suggested Massage Oil Blend:
A warming formula for muscular aches and pains: 25 ml vegetable base oil, 4 drops sweet Marjoram, 4 drops Coriander, 2 drops Juniper berry.

Considerations:
Avoid skin applications during pregnancy. There are no significant reports of adverse skin reactions to sweet Marjoram oil. This oil is not to be confused with the less expensive Spanish Marjoram (*Thymus mastichina*) which, as the botanical name confirms, is actually a species of Thyme and therefore has a different chemical composition (refer to the previous profile).

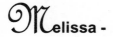elissa -

Melissa officinalis

Synonym: Lemon balm

Plant Family: Lamiaceae (Labiatae)

Note   Top to middle
Odour Intensity   Very high

Description:
A bushy perennial herb with bright green serrated leaves and tiny white or pink flowers. The plant is native to the Mediterranean region, though cultivated in many other parts of the world.

The oil is extracted by steam distillation of the leaves and flowering tops. It is a pale yellow liquid with a light, fresh, Lemony aroma. Its odour effect is uplifting, calming and yet also restorative.

Aromatherapy Uses:
Melissa is helpful for cold sores, coughs, bronchitis, indigestion, nausea, irregular menstrual cycle, insomnia, migraine, anxiety, nervous exhaustion and stress-related states.

Aesthetic Blending Guide:
Melissa blends well with citrus oils, Chamomile (especially Roman), Lavender, Petitgrain, Neroli, Geranium, Rose. The oil is highly odoriferous, so use sparingly.

Suggested Massage Oil Blend:
To help soothe nervous tension and anxiety: 25 ml vegetable base oil, 2 drops Melissa, 2 drops Neroli (or Petitgrain), 5 drops Mandarin.

Considerations:
Melissa is a very expensive oil, akin to the price of Rose Otto. This is because the plant yields a very low concentration of essential oil. Therefore, it can be difficult to obtain the genuine product. Many of the so-called Melissa oils on the market are blends of cheaper oils such as Lemon, Lemongrass and Citronella, sometimes with the addition of synthetic chemicals. Reconstituted versions should be labelled as such, and cost infinitely less than genuine Melissa oil. To better enable detection of a mislabelled product, it is essential to become acquainted with the aroma of true Melissa oil and to compare it with various reconstituted versions. However, true Melissa is a relatively new oil to aromatherapy and has not been thoroughly tested for safety on human skin. Available data indicates that the oil can irritate sensitive skin. Always use in the lowest recommended concentrations.

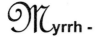yrrh -

Commiphora myrrha

Plant Family: Burseraceae

Note   Base
Odour Intensity   Very high

Other Species:
There are two principal species of *Commiphora* which are used for essential oil production: African or Somali (*C. molmol*) and Arabian or Yemen Myrrh (*C. abyssinica*).

Description:
The plant is native to the Middle East, North Africa and Northern India.

The oil is extracted by steam distillation of myrrh 'tears' (the little pieces of solidified oleo gum resin which exude through natural fissures in the bark of this small tree or shrub and harden on contact with the air). The distilled oil is a pale amber, slightly viscous substance with a warm, balsamic, slightly medicinal aroma. The odour effect is head-clearing, decongestant and warming.

Aromatherapy Uses:
Athlete's foot, arthritic pain, chapped and cracked skin, ringworm, wounds, bronchitis, catarrh, coughs, gingivitis and other gum disorders, mouth ulcers, sore throat, laryngitis, indigestion, delayed periods outside pregnancy (reputedly), thrush, colds and 'flu.

Aesthetic Blending Guide:
Myrrh is not an easy oil to blend. Unless used in very small quantities, the tenacious aroma will predominate your blends. Nevertheless, it can work well with Benzoin, Cypress, Frankincense, Juniper (berry or needle), Lavender, Orange, Palmarosa, Pine, Geranium, Patchouli, Thymes, mints, Ginger, Coriander, Cinnamon, Lemongrass and Sandalwood.

Suggested Massage Oil Blend:
To help ease arthritic pain: also as a chest rub for respiratory ailments: 25 ml vegetable base oil, 3 drops Myrrh, 3 drops Juniper berry, 4 drops Frankincense.

Considerations:
It is essential that you purchase the *essential oil* of Myrrh, not Myrrh resinoid. The latter is a sticky substance, solidifying with age, captured by means of volatile solvents. To make it more parable, it is sometimes diluted with di-ethyl phthalate - a substance which has recently been branded as potentially carcinogenic. So do ask the right questions of your supplier! Myrrh is also tentatively regarded as an emmenagogue (a substance capable of promoting menstruation), so it is best avoided during pregnancy.

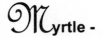**yrtle -**   *Myrtus communis*

Plant Family: Myrtaceae

Note   Middle
Odour Intensity Medium to high

Description:
A small tree with small, sharp-pointed leaves and white flowers, followed by small black berries.   Myrtle is Native to north Africa, but cultivated extensively in the Mediterranean region.

The oil is extracted by steam distillation of the leaves and twigs. It is a yellowish-Orange liquid with a fresh, camphoraceous aroma, akin to Eucalyptus but sweeter and less piercing. Its odour effect is head-clearing and refreshing.

Aromatherapy Uses:
Helpful for acne, oily skin, bronchitis, catarrh, coughs, colds and 'flu, and as a fumigant when infectious illness is around.

Aesthetic Blending Guide:
Myrtle blends well with Bergamot, Grapefruit, Lemon, Clary Sage, Hyssop, Bay, Lavandin, Lavender, Cardomom, Ginger, Clove, Coriander, Ravensara.

Suggested Bath Oil Blend:
To ease cold and 'flu symptoms: 4 drops myrtle, 1 drop Cardomom, 3 drops Lavender. The same combination and quantity of oils can be blended with 20 ml vegetable base oil and applied as a chest rub.

Considerations:
Sensible precautions apply as with all concentrated essential oils. Refer to Essential Oil Safety Precautions pages 17 and 18.

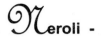eroli -

Citrus aurantium var. amara

Plant Family: Rutaceae

Note   Middle
Odour Intensity   Medium

Other Species: The essence is also extracted from *C. aurantium* var. *dulcis* or *C. aurantium* subsp. *aurantium.*

Description:
The fruit of the bitter orange tree is earth-shaped, a little rougher and darker than the sweet orange. Like other citrus trees, the bitter orange is native to Asia, though cultivated extensively in the Mediterranean region.

The oil is captured by steam distillation of freshly picked Orange blossom. Orange flower water is a by-product of the distillation process. It is also possible to obtain a solvent extracted version of Neroli, which is commonly labelled 'Orange Flower Absolute'. The oil is a pale yellow liquid, becoming darker with age, with a light, sweet-floral fragrance. The absolute is dark brown and viscous with a fresh, sweet-floral fragrance, more akin to that of the fresh plant material. The odour effect of both the absolute and the essential oil is uplifting and soothing: a reputed aphrodisiac.

Aromatherapy Uses:
Skin care (most skin types), as a preventative of stretch marks, palpitations, poor circulation, diarrhoea, pre-menstrual syndrome, mild depression, nervous tension and other stress related states.

Aesthetic Blending Guide:
Neroli blends well with many oils, especially Benzoin, Cedarwood, citrus essences, Chamomile (Roman), Clary Sage, Coriander, Frankincense, Geranium, Jasmine, Lavender, Petitgrain, Rose, Rosemary, Ylang Ylang.

Suggested Bath Oil Blend:
To revive your spirits after a period of prolonged stress: 3 drops Neroli,1 drop Coriander, 1 drop Lavender, 1 drop Geranium (or Rosemary).

Considerations:
Sensible precautions apply as with all concentrated essential oils. Refer to Essential Oil Safety Precautions pages 17 and 18.

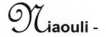iaouli -

Melaleuca viridiflora

Plant Family: Myrtaceae

Note   Top
Odour Intensity   High

Description:
An evergreen tree with tapering leaves, a flexible trunk, spongy bark and bearing spikes of yellowish flowers. Niaouli is native to Australia.

The oil is extracted by steam distillation of the leaves and young twigs. Niaouli oil must also be rectified (re-distilled) to remove irritant aldehydes. The oil is a yellowish or greenish liquid with a fresh camphoraceous aroma. Its odour effect is invigorating and head-clearing.

Aromatherapy Uses:
Acne, boils, burns, wounds, insect bites and stings, muscular aches and pains, rheumatic pain, poor circulation, haemorrhoids, varicose veins, bronchitis, colds and 'flu, coughs, sore throat. Niaouli is being used in some hospitals to help prevent burning of the skin caused by radiotherapy.

Aesthetic Blending Guide:
Niaouli blends well with Lemon, Lavandin, Lavender, Clary Sage, Rosemary, Pine, Geranium, Sweet Marjoram.

Suggested Vaporising Blend:
An invigorating blend to facilitate clarity of thought: it can also be used to disinfect the air when infectious illness is around: 4 drops Niaouli, 4 drops Pine (any variety according to aroma preference), 6 drops Lemon.

Considerations:
Although generally regarded as non-toxic and non-irritant, it is vital to obtain the oil from a reputable supplier as it is often subject to adulteration.

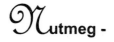utmeg -

Myristica fragrans

Plant Family: Myristicaceae

Note   Middle
Odour Intensity   Very high

Description:
A tropical evergreen tree native to the Moluccas and the West Indies.

The oil is extracted by steam distillation of the crushed Nutmegs.
It is exported from the West Indies and Molucca Islands, then re-distilled in France to improve the quality. An oil can also be obtained from the dried aril or mace (which surrounds the nutmeg), but this is rarely available for aromatherapy or perfumery. More often, the arils are removed from the Nutmegs and then sold for culinary purposes. Nutmeg oil is pale yellow with a sweet and spicy aroma. Its odour effect is warming and comforting: a reputed aphrodisiac.

Aromatherapy Uses:
Arthritic and rheumatic pain, muscular aches and pains, poor circulation, indigestion, flatulence, neuralgia, nervous exhaustion.

Aesthetic Blending Guide:
Nutmeg blends well with citrus oils, Coriander, Geranium, Rosemary, Neroli, Lavender, Lavandin, Bay, Petitgrain, Rose, Ylang Ylang. The oil is highly odoriferous, so use sparingly.

Suggested Vaporising Blend:
A rich, fruity blend ideal as a room perfume at Christmas: 1 drop Nutmeg, 3 drops Orange, 1 drop Coriander, 2 drops Bergamot, 1 drop Neroli.

Considerations:
Nutmeg is a very powerful oil, and thus usually sold as a 'restricted' product solely for professional use. Overuse of the oil (or the whole spice) can cause nausea, hallucinations, over-rapid heartbeat and eventually stupor. It may also irritate sensitive skin, so always use in the lowest recommended concentrations, or use it solely as a room scent. Avoid during pregnancy.

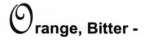range, Bitter -

Citrus aurantium var. amara

Plant Family: Rutaceae

Note   Top
Odour Intensity   Medium

Description:
An evergreen tree with dark green glossy leaves and fragrant white flowers. The fruits are smaller and darker than the sweet orange. The tree is native to Asia, though cultivated extensively in the Mediterranean.

The oil is extracted by cold expression of the outer peel of the almost ripe fruit. It is a yellowish-Orange liquid with a fresh, somewhat sharp, citrusy aroma. Its odour effect is uplifting and refreshing.

Aromatherapy Uses:
Although Bitter Orange oil shares the properties of Sweet Orange, it is not commonly used for aromatherapy massage (see Considerations). However, its perfume is generally preferred for perfumery purposes: it also makes a wonderful room scent (blended with other compatible oils) to help alleviate mild depression.

Aesthetic Blending Guide:
Bitter Orange oil blends well with other citrus oils, and with Jasmine, Neroli, Ylang Ylang, Cedarwood, Sandalwood, Frankincense, Ciste, Coriander (and other spices), Lavender, Lavandin, Rosemary, Vetiver.

Suggested Vaporising Blend:
A joyful harmony: 4 drops Bitter Orange, 2 drops Neroli, 1 drop Rosemary.

Considerations:
Do not use on sensitive skin. For normal skin, it's best used in very low concentration blended with other compatible oils. In this author's opinion, however, it is best to err on the side of caution and avoid skin applications. For the oil is strongly phototoxic and is likely to provoke unsightly patches of hyper-pigmentation if applied shortly before exposure to simulated or natural sunlight. Any substance capable of weakening the skin's resistance to ultra violet light may contribute to the development of skin cancer in individuals predisposed to the condition. Avoid during pregnancy.

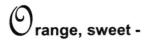range, sweet - *Citrus sinensis*

Plant Family: Rutaceae

Note   Top
Odour Intensity   Medium

Description:
An evergreen green tree with glossy leaves and fragrant white flowers, followed by the fruits. The tree is native to Asia, though extensively cultivated in the Mediterranean region and the USA. Brazil is the largest single producer of the oil, followed by Florida then many smaller sources throughout the world.

The oil is extracted by cold expression of the rind of the fruit. An inferior grade essential oil can be steam distilled from the fruit pulp, which contains oil bearing peel fragments. Overall Orange essential oil is a by-product of Orange juice manufacture. The expressed oil is yellowy-Orange with a sweet and refreshing aroma. The distilled version has a paler yellow hue and lacks the fresh-smelling top notes found in the expressed oil. The odour effect of orange essence (the expressed oil in particular) is uplifting and cheery.

Aromatherapy Uses:
Palpitations, bronchitis, colds and 'flu, indigestion, mild depression, nervous tension and other stress-related states.

Aesthetic Blending Guide:
Sweet Orange essence blends well with other citrus essences, Basil, Clary Sage, Coriander, Ginger, Cinnamon, Clove bud, Frankincense, Geranium, Lavender, Lavandin, Myrrh, Neroli, Patchouli, Rosemary.

Suggested Massage Oil Blend:
A warming, mood-elevating formula: 25 ml vegetable base oil, 4 drops Sweet Orange, 1 drop Nutmeg, 3 drops Petitgrain, 1 drop Rosemary.

Considerations:
Some reports suggest that both the expressed and distilled oils are phototoxic: other studies indicate otherwise. It appears that the oil extracted from the Bitter Orange (*C. aurantium* var. *amara*) is much more likely to provoke photosensitivity. Nevertheless, it is advisable to err on the side of caution by avoiding skin applications of Sweet Orange oil shortly before exposure to natural or simulated sunlight. Certainly, the oil can irritate sensitive skin, especially if used in concentrations above 1%. The potential of all citrus oils to cause skin irritation and sensitisation increases once the oil begins to oxidise. Orange essence deteriorates very quickly, so it is best to use it up within six months of opening the bottle.

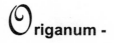**riganum -**   *Origanum vulgare*

Plant Family: Lamiaceae (Labiatae)

Note   Middle
Odour Intensity   Very high

Description:
The essential oil known as 'oreganum' is extracted from the herb commonly known as oregano. It is a bushy perennial with small pinkish-red flowers. Oregano is native to Europe, though now cultivated throughout the world.

The oil is captured by steam distillation of the dried flowering tops of the herb. It is a yellowish liquid, becoming darker with age, with a strong, herbaceous-camphoraceous aroma. Its odour effect is generally perceived as warming and stimulating.

Aromatherapy Uses:
Not recommended for home use (see Considerations). If used professionally, helpful for muscular aches and pains, tennis elbow. It can also be used as a fumigant.

Aesthetic Blending Guide:
Origanum blends well with Lavender, Pine, Rosemary, Cedarwood.

Suggested Vaporising Blend:
As a fumigant when infectious illness is around: 4 drops Origanum 4 drops Rosemary, 4 drops Pine.

Considerations:
Origanum is usually sold as a restricted oil, solely for professional use. Although a marvellous bactericidal and anti-viral agent, it can be harmful to the skin and mucous membranes if used without proper knowledge. The home user is advised never to apply the oil to skin, no matter how diluted. Never use in steam inhalations. Avoid during pregnancy. However, the oil may be used cautiously by the home user as a fumigant (see Suggested Vaporising Blend).

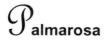almarosa

Cymbopogon martinii

Plant Family: Gramineae

Note   Middle
Odour Intensity   Very high

Description:
An aromatic grass closely related to lemongrass, citronella and vetiver. Although native to India, palmarosa is extensively cultivated in Africa, Madagascar, Indonesia and the Comoros Islands.

The oil is extracted by steam distillation of the fresh or dried grass. It is a yellowish-green liquid with a strong, sweet, Geranium-like aroma, but with an earthy undertone. Its odour effect is uplifting and stimulating.

Aromatherapy Uses:
Skin care (especially oily or dehydrated skin), acne, boils, wounds, loss of appetite, digestive upsets, feverish conditions, nervous exhaustion and other stress-related states.

Aesthetic Blending Guide:
Palmarosa blends well with Cedarwood, citrus essences, Chamomile (Roman), Clary Sage, Coriander, Geranium, Lavender, Lavandin, Patchouli, Petitgrain, Sandalwood. The oil is highly odoriferous, so use sparingly.

Suggested Bath Oil Blend:
A restorative harmony for helping to alleviate the effects of prolonged stress: 2 drops Palmarosa, 3 drops Clary Sage, 2 drops Coriander.

Considerations:
Generally regarded as non-irritant to skin, but only if used in low concentrations of around 1%.

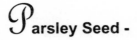 **arsley Seed -**   *Petroselinum sativum*

Plant Family: Apiaceae (Umbelliferae)

Note   Middle
Odour Intensity   Medium to high

Description:
A biennial herb with crinkly bright green leaves, producing umbels of greenish-yellow flowers in the second year of growth. The small brownish seeds are sickle-shaped. Parsley is native to the Mediterranean region, but now cultivated world-wide.

The oil is extracted by steam distillation of the ripe seed. It is a pale amber or brownish liquid with a woody-spicy, herbaceous aroma. Its odour effect is generally perceived as warming and restorative.

Aromatherapy Uses:
A detoxifying oil, helpful for cellulite, arthritis, rheumatism and sciatica. Also for colic, indigestion, delayed periods outside pregnancy, painful periods, to assist childbirth, cystitis, nervous exhaustion.

Aesthetic Blending Guide:
Not recommended for unsupervised home use, except perhaps as a Vaporising oil (see Considerations). Parsley seed oil blends well with Clary Sage, Coriander, Carrot seed, Cumin, Clary Sage, Neroli, Petitgrain, Rose. The oil is highly odoriferous, so use sparingly.

Suggested Vaporising Blend:
An unusual, restorative aroma to help alleviate nervous exhaustion: 2 drops parsley seed, 3 drops Clary Sage, 2 drops Coriander.

Considerations:
Usually sold as a restricted oil, solely for professional use. However, it may be used sparingly to perfume a room (see Suggested Vaporising Blend).

The oil is classified as moderately toxic and may irritate the skin. Use in moderation. Avoid during pregnancy.

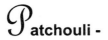atchouli -

Pogostemon cablin

Plant Family: Lamiaceae (Labiatae)

Note   Base
Odour Intensity   Very high

Description:
An herbaceous plant with soft 'furry' leaves and white flowers tinged with purple. Patchouli is native to Malaysia, but cultivated in India, China and South America. 90% of the world supply comes from Sumatra (a large island in the Indonesian group of islands).

The oil is extracted by steam distillation of the dried fermented leaves. It is a dark amber viscous liquid with an extremely tenacious, earthy-musky aroma, which becomes sweeter as the harsh top notes begin to wane. Unlike most other essential oils, Patchouli improves with age. Its odour effect is warming and restorative: a reputed aphrodisiac.

Aromatherapy Uses:
Skin and hair care (especially oily skin and scalp conditions), abscesses, acne, athlete's foot, bed sores, cracked and sore skin, dandruff, weeping eczema, as an insect repellent, wounds, mild depression, nervous exhaustion and other stress-related states.

Aesthetic Blending Guide:
Patchouli blends well with Bergamot (and other citrus essences), Cedarwood, Clary Sage, Clove bud, Lavender, Myrrh, Geranium, Palmarosa, Petitgrain, Rose, Neroli, Sandalwood, Vetiver. The oil is highly odoriferous, so use sparingly.

Suggested Massage Oil Blend:
A tenacious blend with a masculine character. Helpful for nervous exhaustion - and perhaps as a warming aphrodisiac! 25 ml vegetable base oil, 2 drops Patchouli, 1 drop Ginger, 2 drops Palmarosa, 4 drops Mandarin.

Considerations:
Sensible precautions apply as with all concentrated essential oils. Refer to Essential Oil Safety Precautions pages 17 and 18.

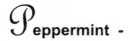eppermint -

Mentha piperita

Plant Family: Lamiaceae (Labiatae)

Note   Top to middle
Odour Intensity Very high

Description:
A spreading herb with dark green leaves and violet flowers. Peppermint is native to the Mediterranean and Western Asia. The main production area is the USA, followed by India.

China is also a big producer of Peppermint mint oil, but this is a different species (*Mentha arvensis*), often referred to as Chinese Peppermint or Corn Mint. Commercial supplies however, are usually fractionated to remove most of the menthol content, thus *Mentha piperita* is a more appropriate oil for aromatherapy.

The oil is extracted by steam distillation of the whole plant (excepting the roots which are left to produce subsequent crops). Harvest takes place just before full bloom. The oil is a pale yellow liquid with a fresh, piercing and minty aroma. Its odour effect is awakening, cooling and head-clearing.

Aromatherapy Uses:
Bruises, sprains and strains, swellings, ringworm, scabies, toothache, neuralgia, muscular aches and pains, bronchitis, offensive breath, sinusitis, spasmodic cough, colic, indigestion, irritable bowel syndrome (oil taken internally in the form of Peppermint capsules - dosage according to the manufacturer's instructions), flatulence, mouth ulcers, mouth thrush, nausea, feverish conditions, colds and 'flu, fainting, headache, mental fatigue, migraine.

Aesthetic Blending Guide:
Peppermint blends well with Benzoin, Clary Sage, Eucalyptus, Geranium, Lavender, Lemon, Marjoram, Rosemary. The oil is highly odoriferous, so use sparingly.

Suggested Vaporising Blend:
A cooling blend for sultry summer days: 1 drop Peppermint, 2 drops Clary Sage, 2 drops Lavender, 2 drops Lemon.

Considerations:
Use well diluted as it may irritate the skin. It is also advisable to avoid skin applications during pregnancy.

NB.
Never use on babies and young children as the oil may cause breathing problems.

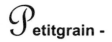**etitgrain -**   Citrus aurantium var. amara,

                                    also   C. aurantium subsp. aurantium

Plant Family: Rutaceae

Note   Top to middle
Odour Intensity   Medium to high

Description:
The tree is native to Asia, though now cultivated in North Africa, Paraguay and the Mediterranean.

The oil is captured by steam distillation of the leaves and twigs of the bitter orange tree. It is a pale yellow liquid with a fresh, woody-herbaceous aroma reminiscent of Neroli but much less refined. The odour effect is cooling and uplifting.

Aromatherapy Uses:
Skin and hair care (oily), indigestion, insomnia, pre-menstrual syndrome, nervous exhaustion and other stress-related states.

Aesthetic Blending Guide:
Petitgrain blends well with Bergamot (and other citrus oils), Benzoin, Cedarwood, Clary Sage, Clove, Coriander, Cypress, Frankincense, Geranium, Lavender, Neroli, Palmarosa, parsley seed, Rose, Rosemary, Vetiver.

Suggested Massage Blend:
A gentle restorative to soothe a jangled nervous system: 25 ml vegetable base oil, 3 drops Petitgrain, 1 drop Celery seed, 2 drops Pine, 2 drops Lavender.

Considerations:
Sensible precautions apply as with all concentrated essential oils. Refer to Essential Oil Safety Precautions pages 17 and 18.

$\mathcal{P}$ine, Scots -

Pinus sylvestris

Plant Family: Pinaceae

Note   Top to middle
Odour Intensity   Medium to high

Description:
A tall evergreen conifer with a flat crown and reddish-brown, deeply fissured bark. The tree is native to northern Europe.

The oil is extracted by steam distillation of the Pine needles. An inferior grade oil is also extracted from the cones, twigs and wood chippings, but this is not recommended for Aromatherapy. The oil is a colourless to pale yellow liquid. The aroma is turpentine-like with a camphoraceous undertone. Its odour effect is refreshing, cooling and restorative.

Aromatherapy Uses:
Cuts and abrasions, wounds, headlice, scabies, excessive perspiration, arthritic and rheumatic pain, gout, muscular aches and pains, poor circulation, asthma (under professional supervision), bronchitis, catarrh, colds and 'flu, coughs, sinusitis, sore throat, cystitis, neuralgia, nervous exhaustion and other stress-related states.

Aesthetic Blending Guide:
Pine blends well with Bergamot (and other citrus oils), Cedarwood, Cypress, Eucalyptus, Frankincense, Juniper, Lavender, Niaouli, Rosemary, Tea Tree, Eucalyptus, Marjoram.

Suggested Massage Oil Blend:
For arthritic and rheumatic pain and to ease the discomfort of overworked muscles: 25 ml vegetable base oil, 4 drops Pine, 2 drops Juniper berry, 4 drops Rosemary.

Considerations:
Generally regarded as non-irritant, although there are reports indicating that the oil is a sensitising agent. Oils which are old and oxidised (chemically altered as a result of exposure to oxygen in the air) are much more likely to cause skin reactions. The oil should be avoided by those with sensitive skin. Always use in the lowest recommended concentrations.

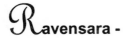avensara -

Ravensara aromatica

Plant Family: Lauraceae

Note   Top
Odour Intensity   High

Description:
The essential oil is extracted by steam distillation of the leaves of a tropical tree native to Madagascar. It has a fresh, camphoraceous aroma with a spicy undertone. The odour effect is generally perceived as warming and revitalising.

Aromatherapy Uses:
Coughs, colds and 'flu, bronchitis, sinusitis, muscular aches and pains, nervous fatigue, mild depression.

Aesthetic Blending Guide:
Ravensara blends well with Bay, Cedarwood, Coriander, Cypress, Eucalyptus, Helichrysum, Lavender, myrtle, Peppermint, Rosemary.

Suggested Massage Oil:
For muscular aches and pains: 25 ml vegetable base oil, 5 drops Ravensara, 3 drops Lavender, 3 drops Rosemary.

Considerations:
There is no traditional therapeutic use of Ravensara oil. Historically, the seeds (known as 'Madagascar Cloves' or Madagascar Nutmeg') have been used as a spice and the bark used in rum-making. Infusions of the leaves are traditionally regarded as a digestive tonic. The therapeutic properties of the oil have not been thoroughly investigated. Most of the information given here is gleaned from anecdotal evidence. Although often cited as 'non-toxic', it should be mentioned that Ravensara oil has never undergone formal testing on humans. Therefore, it should be used in moderation and avoided by pregnant women, elderly people and young children.

$\mathcal{R}$ose Maroc Absolute - *Rosa centifolia* and *R. damascena*

Plant Family: Rosaceae

Note   Middle
Odour Intensity   Medium

Description:
The rose is believed to have originated in Persia, though now cultivated throughout the world. The intensely fragrant varieties used for oil production have masses of pale pink or rosy-purple flowers.

The Absolute is captured by solvent extraction of the fresh petals. It is a yellowy-Orange viscous liquid with a sweet, mellow fragrance. Its odour effect is warming, soothing and gently uplifting: a reputed aphrodisiac.

Aromatherapy Uses:
Skin care (most skin types), to help reduce thread veins, palpitations, nausea, mild depression, insomnia, headache, pre-menstrual syndrome, nervous tension and other stress-related states.

Aesthetic Blending Guide:
Rose absolute blends well with a broad spectrum of other oils, including Bergamot (and other citrus oils), Benzoin, Cedarwood, Chamomile (Roman), Clary Sage, Frankincense, Geranium, Jasmine (and other floral absolutes) Neroli, Sandalwood, Petitgrain, Lavender, Patchouli, Clove (and other spices), Palmarosa, Ylang Ylang.

Suggested Perfume Blend:
A voluptuous floriental blend - strictly not for the faint hearted! 5 ml Jojoba   , 8 drops Rose absolute, 3 drops Coriander, 4 drops Mandarin, 4 drops Ylang Ylang complete.

Considerations:
Generally regarded as non-irritant, non-sensitising and the least toxic of all absolutes. However, when used in high concentration (for example, as a skin perfume) it may irritate sensitive skin. For therapeutic purposes, many Aromatherapists favour the more costly *distilled* Rose Otto because its extraction does not involve the use of petro-chemical derived solvents.

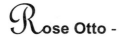**ose Otto -** *R. damascena* and several other varieties of <u>Rosa</u>

Plant Family: Rosaceae

Note   Middle to base
Odour Intensity   High

Description:
The Damask rose (*R. damascena*) is a small prickly shrub, with delicately pink blooms and whitish hairy leaves (see also Rose Maroc).

The oil is extracted by steam distillation of the fresh petals. It is a virtually colourless liquid which becomes semi-solid at cool temperatures. The aroma is sweet and mellow with a hint of Cloves and vanilla. Its odour effect is warming, soothing and heady: a reputed aphrodisiac.

Aromatherapy Uses:
Skin care (most skin types, especially mature), conjunctivitis (Rosewater), to help reduce thread veins, eczema, palpitations, hay fever, poor circulation, asthma (under professional supervision), coughs, cold sores, irregular menstruation, heavy menstruation, pre-menstrual syndrome, mild depression, insomnia, headache, nervous tension and other stress-related states.

Aesthetic Blending Guide:
If the oil is semi-solid, roll the bottle between your hands for a minute or two and it will become liquid. As with Rose absolute, Rose Otto blends well with a broad spectrum of essential oils, especially other florals, spices, woods, resins and citrus oils. The oil is highly odoriferous and can be used in tiny amounts to create pleasing blends of good tenacity.

Suggested Massage Blend:
A sensuous blend to reduce stress levels and promote a sense of well-being: 25 ml vegetable base oil, 1 drop Rose Otto, 3 drops Sandalwood, 1 drop Coriander, 3 drops Bergamot.

Considerations:
Sensible precautions apply as with all concentrated essential oils. Refer to Essential Oil Safety Precautions pages 17 and 18.

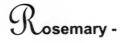 **osemary -** *Rosmarinus officinalis*

Plant Family: Lamiaceae (Labiatae)

Note   Top to middle
Odour Intensity   Medium to high

Description:
A shrubby evergreen bush with silvery-green needle-shaped leaves and pale blue flowers. Rosemary is native to the Mediterranean, though now cultivated world-wide.

The oil is extracted by steam distillation of the flowering tops. Inferior grade oils are distilled from the whole plant. The top grade oil is a colourless to pale yellow liquid with a woody-balsamic, camphoraceous aroma. Lower quality oils are highly camphoraceous (like Eucalyptus) and somewhat harsh. The odour effect is refreshing and head-clearing, and yet warming and restorative.

Aromatherapy Uses:
Skin and hair care (oily), dandruff, to promote growth of healthy hair, headlice, as an insect repellent, scabies, colds and 'flu, bronchitis, coughs, muscular aches and pains, arthritic and rheumatic pain, poor circulation, painful menstruation, headaches, mental fatigue, neuralgia, depression, nervous exhaustion and other stress-related states.

Aesthetic Blending Guide:
Rosemary blends well with Basil, Cedarwood, Coriander and other spice oils, citrus essences, Frankincense, Geranium, Lemongrass, Lavender, Peppermint, Petitgrain, Pine, Thyme.

Suggested Bath Blend:
An enlivening and restorative formula: 4 drops Rosemary, 1 drop Lemongrass, 1 drop Cardomom.

Considerations:
Avoid skin applications during pregnancy. There is a remote chance that the oil may trigger an epileptic seizure in those predisposed to the condition. Rosemary oil may irritate sensitive skin.

$\mathcal{S}$andalwood (AGMARK grade) - _Santalum album_

Plant Family: Santalaceae

Note   Base
Odour Intensity Low

Description:
A semi-parasitic tree which grows on the roots of neighbouring trees during the first seven years of its life. Native to tropical Asia, including Mysore in India.

The oil is extracted by steam distillation of the roots and heartwood of the tree, which is native to India. The oil is pale yellow and viscous, with a soft, sweet-woody, balsamic aroma of excellent tenacity. Its odour effect is usually perceived as soothing and deeply relaxing: reputedly aphrodisiac.

NB:
In India, the government has given the term AGMARK (Agricultural Guarantee Mark) to their Sandalwood oil. This confirms that it is a pure unadulterated essential oil captured from the species commonly known as 'Mysore Sandalwood'.

Aromatherapy Uses:
Skin care (acne, dry, oily), bronchitis, catarrh, coughs, laryngitis, sore throat, diarrhoea, nausea, cystitis, mild depression, insomnia, nervous tension and other stress-related states.

Aesthetic Blending Guide:
Sandalwood blends well with many other oils, especially Rose, Ylang Ylang, Jasmine, Lavender, Clove, Bergamot, Clary Sage, Geranium, Ciste, Benzoin, Vetiver, Patchouli, Frankincense, Pine, Myrrh.

Suggested Massage Oil Blend:
A relaxing 'masculine' blend: 25 ml vegetable base oil, 4 drops Sandalwood, 1 drop Frankincense, 2 drops Clary Sage, 2 drops Benzoin.

Considerations:
Mysore Sandalwood oil is especially vulnerable to adulteration. Vast quantities are used by the perfume industry, and thus world supplies are often depleted. Occasionally, the oil known as West Indian Sandalwood (Amyris balsamifera) is sold as an inexpensive alternative to Mysore Sandalwood. West Indian Sandalwood oil (also commonly known as Amyris) bears no relation to true Sandalwood oil, having an inferior musky-woody aroma of poor tenacity. Moreover, amyris essential oil should be regarded as potentially risky, for it has not undergone formal testing on humans.

105

$\mathcal{S}$avory, Summer -

Satureja hortensis

Plant Family: Lamiaceae (Labiatae)

Note   Top to middle
Odour Intensity   High

Description:
An annual herb with long, slender leaves and tiny mauve flowers. The plant is native to Europe, though extensively cultivated in the USA for its essential oil, which extracted by steam distillation of the whole dried herb. The oil is colourless to pale yellow liquid with a fresh, herbaceous, spicy aroma. Its odour effect is warming and stimulating.

Aromatherapy Uses:
Little used in aromatherapy, and certainly not recommended for home use, except perhaps as a Vaporising oil (see Considerations). French aromatherapy doctors prescribe the oil internally for chronic respiratory ailments and intestinal parasites. The oil's powerful antibacterial properties make it an excellent ingredient in fumigant blends.

Aesthetic Blending Guide:
When used as a fumigant, summer savory blends well with Pine, Rosemary, Lavender, Lavandin, Lemon.

Suggested Vaporising Blend:
As a fumigant when infectious illness is around: 3 drops summer savory, 3 drops Pine, 4 drops Lemon.

Considerations:
Usually sold as a restricted oil, solely for professional use. Do not use in steam inhalations, as it is a mucous membrane irritant. Best to avoid skin applications of the oil (no matter how diluted) as it can be highly irritant. Avoid during pregnancy.

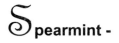

Spearmint -

Mentha spicata

Plant Family: Lamiaceae (Labiatae)

Note   Top to middle
Odour Intensity   Very high

Description:
A hardy perennial herb with bright green lance-shaped leaves and spikes of pink or lilac-coloured flowers. Spearmint is native to the Mediterranean region, though now cultivated in many other parts of the world.

The oil is extracted by steam distillation of the whole plant (excepting the roots which are left to produce subsequent crops). Harvest takes place just before full bloom. The oil is a yellowish-green liquid with a sweet-herbaceous, minty aroma. Its odour effect is cooling, refreshing and invigorating.

Aromatherapy Uses:
Helpful for catarrh, bronchitis, sinusitis, flatulence, nausea, colds and 'flu, headaches, muscular aches and pains, migraine, nervous tension, and as an ingredient in mouthwashes to sweeten the breath.

Aesthetic Blending Guide:
Spearmint blends well with Peppermint, Lavender, Lavandin, Eucalyptus, Rosemary, Basil.

Suggested Steam Inhalation Blend:
To help loosen catarrh and clear blocked sinuses: 1 drop spearmint, 1 drop Rosemary, 1 drop Lavender. Add the oils to a bowl of steaming water (2-3 pt capacity), then cover your head and the bowl with a towel to form a 'tent'. Inhale for 5 minutes.

Considerations:
Generally regarded as non irritant. However, the oil is highly odoriferous and may irritate sensitive skin. Use in the lowest recommended concentrations.

agete -   *Tagetes minuta*

Synonyms: Tagette, tagetes,
                                                     Mexican marigold

Plant Family: Asteraceae (Compositae)

Note   Middle to base
Odour Intensity   Extremely high

NB Many sources wrongly cite this oil as 'Calendula', confusing it with the pot marigold or *Calendula officinalis*.

Description:
A strongly scented annual herb with deeply divided leaves and brownish-orange flowers. Native to South America, but cultivated extensively world wide.

The oil is captured by steam distillation of the fresh flowers and leaves. It is a yellow-Orange, slightly viscous liquid with a bitter-green top note and sweetish undertone. It is difficult to offer a generalised assessment of its odour effect, except to say that it has an offbeat aroma which is loved by some, detested by others.

Aromatherapy Uses:
Not recommended for unsupervised home use, except perhaps as a Vaporising oil (see Considerations). Aromatherapists use it cautiously for treating stubborn cases of athlete's foot, and for ringworm, corns and calluses. The oil reputedly promotes delayed menstruation.

Aesthetic Blending Guide:
Rarely used for its aesthetic qualities. However, a solvent-extracted absolute, with a more pleasing aroma, is produced in small quantities almost exclusively for the perfume industry. The oil is extremely odoriferous and will overpower the aromas of other essential oils. Its aroma has the curious property of becoming stronger when combined with other essential oils. As a Vaporising oil, it's acceptable if mixed with Bergamot, Orange, Lemon or Lavender in very small quantities.

Suggested Vaporising Blend:
A good insect repellent: 1 drop tagetes, 3 drops Lemon, 4 drops Bergamot, 2 drops Lavender.

Considerations:
Usually sold as a 'restricted' oil, solely for professional use. The home user is advised never to the use Tagetes in massage blends, no matter how diluted. It contains quite a high proportion of potentially toxic ketones (mainly tagetone) which may provoke skin reactions. The oil is also phototoxic and may provoke unsightly pigmentation if applied to skin shortly before exposure to simulated or natural sunlight. Avoid during pregnancy.

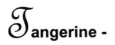**angerine -**   *Citrus reticulata*

Plant Family: Rutaceae

Note   Top
Odour Intensity   Very low

NB
Although the words 'Tangerine' and 'Mandarin' are used interchangeably, they actually denote two slightly different varieties of loose-skinned Orange. The Tangerine is larger and rounder than the Mandarin, with a more yellow skin. Mandarins are grown in the Mediterranean regions of Europe and North Africa: whereas the Tangerine is produced mainly in Texas and Brazil.

Description:
The oil is extracted by cold expression of the outer peel of the fruit. It is an Orange liquid with a fresh, sweet, Orange-like aroma, but having slightly less body than Mandarin. Its odour effect is calming and gently uplifting.

Aromatherapy Uses:
See Mandarin

Aesthetic Blending Guide:
As for Mandarin. It's important to add that both oils have a low Odour Intensity   and usually need to be used in higher than average concentrations, especially when mixed with other oils. Their delicate aromas are easily overpowered.

Suggested Vaporising Oil:
To help promote restful sleep: 6 drops Tangerine, 1 drop Rose Otto (or Rose absolute). The same combination and quantity of oil may be added to the bath water shortly before bedtime.

Considerations:
Although generally regarded as non-toxic and non-irritant, Tangerine oil is slightly phototoxic and may cause uneven pigmentation if applied to skin shortly before exposure to simulated or natural sunlight. The oil also has a relatively short shelf-life, depending on how often the oil is exposed to oxygen in the air. An oxidised oil applied to the skin is likely to cause irritation. It is advisable to use up the oil within 6-9 months of opening the bottle.

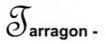arragon -

Artemisia dracunculus

Synonym: Estragon oil

Plant Family: Asteraceae
(Compositae)

Note   Middle
Odour Intensity Very high

Description:
A perennial herb with narrow leaves and tiny yellowish flowers. Tarragon is native to Europe, southern Russia and eastern Asia, though cultivated world-wide.

The oil is extracted by steam distillation of the leaves. It is a yellowish liquid (darkening with age) with a sweet, Aniseed-like top note and green undertone. Its odour effect is warming and stimulating.

Aromatherapy Uses:
Not recommended for unsupervised home use, except perhaps as a Vaporising oil (see Considerations). Professionally it is used for nervous indigestion, PMT, painful periods and absence of periods outside pregnancy.

Aesthetic Blending Guide:
Tarragon blends well with Basil, Ciste, Galbanum, Lavender, Lemon, Orange, Pine. The oil is highly odoriferous, so use sparingly.

Suggested Vaporising Blend:
An interesting blend to help promote good digestion. Vaporise it in the dining room shortly before a rich meal.   Once the meal is served, it is advisable to remove the vaporiser from the room, as the essential oils may compete with the food aromas - that is, unless the corresponding herbs and fruit are used as flavourings!   Recipe: 1 drop tarragon, 2 drops Basil, 3 drops Lemon.

Considerations:
Tarragon oil is quite toxic and is therefore usually sold as a 'restricted' oil, solely for professional use. Do not use on the skin, no matter how diluted. Avoid during pregnancy.

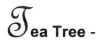ea Tree - _Melaleuca alternifolia_

Plant Family: Myrtaceae

Note   Top
Odour Intensity   High

Description:
A small tree or shrub with needle-like leaves and bottlebrush-like yellow flowers. The tree is native to Australia, from the where the world's supply of tea tree oil is produced.

The oil is extracted by steam distillation of the leaves and twigs. It is a pale yellow liquid with a strong and medicinal aroma reminiscent of a mixture of Juniper and Cypress. The odour effect is cooling and head-clearing.

Aromatherapy Uses:
Acne, athlete's foot, abscesses, cold sores, dandruff, rashes, ringworm, burns, wounds, insect bites and stings, colds and 'flu, catarrh, coughs, veruccae, thrush, cystitis, fevers, as a fumigant when infectious illness is around.

Aesthetic Blending Guide:
Tea Tree does not blend very well with other oils because of its strong, medicinal aroma. However, it is acceptable blended with Eucalyptus, Lemon (and other citrus oils), Lavender, Marjoram, Pine, Rosemary.

Suggested Massage Blend:
A chest rub to ease congestion when suffering from colds and 'flu: 25 ml vegetable base oil, 4 drops Tea Tree, 3 drops Lavender, 3 drops Marjoram Sweet. Apply twice daily.

Considerations:
There are many reports of minor skin reactions caused by continuous use of Tea Tree. Do not use the oil neat or in high concentration for prolonged periods (i.e. upwards of six weeks). For a chronic (long-term) health problem, it is advisable to seek professional advice.

$\mathscr{T}$hyme, Sweet -

Thymus vulgaris

Plant Family: Lamiaceae (Labiatae)

Note   Top
Odour Intensity   High

Description:
A perennial woody herb with greyish-green leaves and pale purple or white flowers. The plant is native to Mediterranean region, though cultivated in other parts of the world.

The oil is extracted by steam distillation of the leaves and flowering tops. It is a pale yellow liquid with a sweet herbaceous aroma. Its odour effect is gently stimulating and warming.

Aromatherapy Uses:
Abscesses, insect bites and stings, scabies, wounds, arthritic and rheumatic pain, gout, muscular aches and pains, asthma (under professional supervision), bronchitis, catarrh, coughs, laryngitis, sinusitis, sore throat, tonsillitis, colds and 'flu, cystitis, as fumigant when infectious illness is around, headaches, nervous exhaustion and other stress-related states.

Aesthetic Blending Guide:
Thyme blends well with Bergamot (and other citrus oils), Lavandin, Lavender, Lemongrass, Melissa, Rosemary, Marjoram, Pine. For massage, baths and steam inhalations it is essential to obtain the correct variety of Thyme oil (see Considerations).

Suggested Bath Blend:
A fortifying mixture to relieve muscular aches and pains, tiredness and mild depression. While the water is running, add 4 tablespoons sea salt (moving water helps to dissolve salt). After the bath is filled, add 3 drops sweet Thyme, 1 drop Lemongrass, 2 drops Rosemary.

Considerations:
Avoid skin applications and steam inhalations during pregnancy. There are many varieties of Thyme oil available, but only a few are gentle enough for the home user. Those oils broadly categorised as 'Red Thyme' are high in potentially caustic phenols such as carvacrol and thymol and should therefore be restricted to professional use. For example, T. Vulgaris cv. thymol.

Those oils which are labelled 'sweet Thyme' are much safer for unsupervised home use because they are high in relatively gentle alcohols such as geraniol and linalol. For example T.vulgaris c.v. linalol. If in doubt, make it clear to your supplier that you require sweet Thyme oil.

Another commonly used oil is labelled 'Wild Thyme' (Thymus serpyllum). Unfortunately, wild plants have very different chemical compositions, even though they may be found growing in the same area. Therefore, unless the oil can be guaranteed non-caustic through GLC analysis, it cannot be guaranteed that a wild Thyme oil will be gentle to skin and mucous membranes.

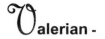**alerian -**   *Valeriana faueriei*

Synonym: *V.officinalis*

Plant Family: Valerianaceae

Note   Base
Odour Intensity   Extremely high

Description:
A perennial herb with deeply divided leaves and many purplish-white flowers. It has a short, thick rhizome, largely showing above ground, which has a strong odour. Valerian is native to Europe and parts of Asia.

The essential oil is captured by steam distillation of the rhizomes. It is an Olive or dark brown liquid (darkening with age) with a penetrating, earthy-musky aroma. Although regarded as a deeply relaxing aroma, its intensity is not appreciated by everyone!

Aromatherapy Uses:
Mainly used blended with other oils for insomnia, nervous indigestion and nervous tension.

Aesthetic Blending Guide:
In this author's opinion, valerian does not blend harmoniously with other oils, for its penetrating odour always predominates, no matter how little is used. Others suggest that it blends well with Cedarwood, Lavender, Patchouli, Pine, Mandarin, Petitgrain, Rosemary and Vetiver. Incidentally, the aroma is much appreciated by cats - especially female cats. Use sparingly!

Suggested Vaporising Blend:
To relax a nervy pussy cat: 1 drop valerian, 5 drops Cedarwood. Please note: cats tend to dislike the aromas of most essential oils, with the exception of valerian, Cedarwood, Sandalwood, Vetiver and Patchouli.

Considerations:
Before attempting to the use the oil, do ensure that the recipient appreciates the aroma. A powerful oil, so always use in the lowest recommended concentrations.

Vetiver -

Vetiveria zizanoides

Plant Family: Poaceae (Gramineae)

Note   Base
Odour Intensity   Very high

Description:
A tall grass with unscented leaves, but highly aromatic roots. The plant is a close relative of other aromatic grasses such as lemongrass and palmarosa. Native to southern India, Indonesia and Sri Lanka, though cultivated in other warm regions.

The essential oil is extracted by steam distillation of the dried and chopped roots of the aromatic grass. The oil is dark brown and viscous with a highly tenacious, earthy, molasses-like aroma. The fragrance improves as the oil ages. Its odour effect is calming and warming: a reputed aphrodisiac.

Aromatherapy Uses:
Skin care (oily), acne, arthritic and rheumatic pain, muscular aches and pains, poor circulation, insomnia, light-headedness (a good 'grounding' essence), pre-menstrual syndrome, mild depression, nervous exhaustion and other stress-related states.

Aesthetic Blending Guide:
Vetiver blends well with Clary Sage, Cedarwood, citrus oils, Jasmine, Lavender, Patchouli, Petitgrain, Mimosa, Neroli, Rose, Sandalwood, Ylang Ylang. The oil is highly odoriferous, so use sparingly.

Suggested Bath Oil Blend:
A deeply relaxing formula reminiscent of a forest floor after rain: 1 drop Vetiver, 1 drop Petitgrain, 2 drops Clary Sage, 2 drops Cedarwood.

Considerations:
Sensible precautions apply as with all concentrated essential oils. Refer to Essential Oil Safety Precautions pages 17 and 18.

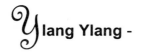lang Ylang -   *Cananga odorata var. genuina*

Plant Family: Annonaceae

Note   Base to middle
Odour Intensity   High

Description:
Ylang ylang (pronounced ee lang ee lang) is a tropical tree with large glossy leaves and intensely fragrant yellow blooms. Most of the oil is produced in Madagascar, Reunion and the Comoros Islands.

The oil is extracted by steam distillation of the fresh flowers. There are several grades of the oil: Ylang Ylang extra, and Ylang Ylang one, two and three. There is also a 'complete' oil.

The extra grade is collected from the first running of the distillation process: the plant material is distilled two or three more times to obtain the lower grades. Ylang Ylang complete represents the total or 'unfractionated' oil which is collected at the end of a long process of distillation. All grades of oil are pale yellow or virtually colourless. The extra and complete grades have a fragrance reminiscent of almonds and Jasmine combined - although Ylang Ylang complete has a lighter, more refined quality. The other fractions are harsh and woody by comparison. Most Aromatherapists favour the more expensive extra and complete grades. The odour effect of a good quality Ylang Ylang is generally perceived as warming and intoxicating: a reputed aphrodisiac.

Aromatherapy Uses:
High blood pressure, palpitations, mild depression, insomnia, pre-menstrual syndrome, nervous tension and other stress-related states.

Aesthetic Blending Guide:
Ylang Ylang blends well with other florals, Black Pepper (and other spices), citrus oils, Frankincense, Geranium, Sandalwood, Vetiver. The oil is highly odoriferous, so use sparingly.

Suggested Massage Blend:
A relaxing and sensuous blend: 25 ml vegetable base oil, 2 drops Ylang Ylang, 3 drops Sandalwood, 2 drops Lime.

Considerations:
Generally regarded as non-irritant. However, it can provoke sensitisation reactions in some people.

QUICK GUIDE TO ESSENTIAL OILS
FOR COMMON AILMENTS

This simple reference is included to help round out the picture. It is not meant to be prescriptive, neither is it by any means comprehensive. Unless you have a good knowledge of natural healing principles and aromatherapy applications, the information will need to be used in conjunction with a more in-depth book on holistic aromatherapy such as one of the publications listed under Suggested Reading, page 124. For general advice on preparing and using essential oils, see Chapter 2.

ACNE
Cedarwood (Virginian or Atlas), chamomile (German or Roman), frankincense, juniper berry, lavender, myrtle, patchouli, rose otto, rosemary, tea tree.

ANXIETY & STRESS
Angelica, basil, bergamot (and other citrus oils), chamomile (German or Roman), clary sage, cypress, frankincense, geranium, ho-leaf, juniper berry, lavender, marjoram (sweet), melissa (true), neroli, nutmeg, patchouli, petitgrain, rose otto, sandalwood, valerian, vetiver, ylang ylang. Also, floral absolutes such as jasmine and rose maroc.

ARTHRITIS & RHEUMATISM
Angelica, birch (white),cedarwood (Virginian or Atlas), celery seed, chamomile (German or Roman), coriander, cypress, eucalyptus, ginger, juniper berry, lavender, marjoram (sweet), pine, rosemary, vetiver.

ATHLETE'S FOOT
Cedarwood (Atlas), eucalyptus, lavender, patchouli, pine, tea tree.

BOILS & ABCESSES
Bergamot FCF, chamomile (preferably German), lavender, marjoram (sweet), lavender, tea tree.

BRONCHITIS
Angelica, cedarwood (Atlas or Virginian), ciste, eucalyptus, frankincense, lavender, peppermint, pine, rose otto, rosemary, sandalwood, spearmint, tea tree.

BRUISES - See 'Sprains and Bruises'

BURNS & SCALDS (minor)
Chamomile (preferably German), eucalyptus, frankincense, lavender, tea tree.

CATARRH
Cedarwood (Atlas or Virginian), eucalyptus, frankincense, ginger, juniper berry, lavender, lemon, marjoram (sweet), myrtle, myrrh, peppermint, pine, rose otto, rosemary, sandalwood, spearmint, tea tree.

CHILBLAINS
Chamomile (preferably German), lavender, marjoram (sweet).

CIRCULATION, POOR
Angelica, Black pepper, coriander, cypress, eucalyptus, geranium, ginger, lavender, marjoram (sweet), neroli, peppermint, pine, rosemary.

COLDS AND FLU

Angelica, cedarwood (Atlas or Virginian), coriander, eucalyptus, ginger, lavender, lemon, marjoram (sweet), myrtle, peppermint, pine, spearmint, tea tree, thyme (sweet).

COLD SORES

Chamomile (German), eucalyptus, melissa (true), tea tree.

COUGHS

Cedarwood (Atlas or Virginian), ciste, cypress, eucalyptus, frankincense, ginger, marjoram (sweet), pine, rosemary, sandalwood, tea tree.

CUTS AND GRAZES

Eucalyptus, lavender, tea tree.

DANDRUFF

Cedarwood (Atlas and Virginian), eucalyptus, lavender, rosemary, tea tree.

DEPRESSION (mild)

Basil, bergamot (and other citrus oils), clary sage, cardomom, coriander, frankincense, geranium, lavender, lemongrass, neroli, patchouli, petitgrain, rose otto, rosemary, sandalwood, ylang ylang. Also, floral absolutes such as jasmine, lime (linden) blossom and rose.

EARACHE

Chamomile (preferably German), lavender, peppermint, rosemary.

FATIGUE AND NERVOUS EXHAUSTION

Angelica, basil, bergamot (and other citrus oils), cardomom, coriander, geranium, ginger, juniper berry, lavender, lemongrass, marjoram (sweet), myrtle, peppermint, pine, rose otto, rosemary, spearmint.

FEVERS

Bergamot FCF, clary sage, eucalyptus, juniper berry, lemon, peppermint, tea tree.

FLUID RETENTION

Massage (particularly the form known as lymphatic drainage massage) is the most effective method, along with oils such as cypress, juniper berry, pine, rosemary.

GINGIVITIS

Eucalyptus, myrrh, tea tree.

HAEMORRHOIDS (to help reduce pain and inflammation)

Cypress, frankincense.

HAYFEVER

Chamomile (preferably German), eucalyptus, pine, rose otto.

HEADACHE

Lavender, marjoram (sweet), peppermint, rose otto, rosemary.

HEADLICE

Eucalyptus, geranium, lavender, pine, rosemary, tea tree.

INDIGESTION AND HEARTBURN

Angelica, basil, cardomom, chamomile (German or Roman), clary sage, coriander, ginger, lavender, marjoram (sweet), neroli, peppermint, spearmint. Heartburn: chamomile (preferably German).

INSECT BITES AND STINGS

Eucalyptus, lavender, tea tree.

INSECT REPELLENTS

Cedarwood (Virginian or Atlas), citronella, eucalyptus, lavender, lemongrass, patchouli, peppermint, rosemary, tea tree.

INSOMNIA

Chamomile (preferably Roman), clary sage, lavender, mandarin, marjoram (sweet), neroli, rose otto, sandalwood, valerian.

LIBIDO (To enhance or restore in stress-related conditions)

Angelica, black pepper, cardomom, clary sage, coriander, ginger, jasmine absolute, neroli, nutmeg, patchouli, rose, rosemary, ylang ylang (all are reputed aphrodisiacs).

MENSTRUAL PROBLEMS:

Loss of periods, scanty or irregular periods:

Angelica, carrot seed, clary sage, juniper berry, marjoram (sweet), rose otto.

Painful periods:

Angelica, carrot seed, chamomile (German or Roman), clary sage, frankincense, hops, juniper berry, lavender, marjoram (sweet), rose otto, rosemary, valerian.

Heavy periods:

Chamomile (German or Roman), geranium, frankincense, cypress, rose otto.

PMS: See oils for Anxiety and Stress, Depression, Fluid Retention

MENOPAUSAL SYMPTOMS Hot flushes, night sweats:

clary sage, cypress (see also Anxiety and Stress, Depression, Mental Fatigue, Migraine)

MENTAL FATIGUE

Angelica, basil, cardomom, coriander, eucalyptus, geranium, lavender, lemongrass, myrtle, peppermint, pine, rosemary, spearmint.

MIGRAINE

Lavender, marjoram (sweet), peppermint, rose otto, rosemary.

MOUTH ULCERS

Myrrh, peppermint, tea tree.

MUSCULAR ACHES AND PAINS

Birch (white), black pepper, chamomile (German or Roman), clary sage, coriander, eucalyptus, frankincense, ginger, juniper berry, lavender, marjoram (sweet), peppermint, pine, rosemary.

NAPPY RASH

In this instance the unsupervised home use of essential oils not recommended. Try macerated calendula oil instead.

NAUSEA (it is essential to choose according to aroma preference)
Ginger, lavender, peppermint, spearmint, sandalwood

NIPPLES - Sore Cracked
In this instance the unsupervised home use of essential oils not recommended. Try macerated calendula oil instead.

PALPITATIONS
Chamomile (German or Roman), lavender, neroli, melissa (true), petitgrain, rose otto, ylang ylang.

RINGWORM
Eucalyptus, lavender, patchouli, peppermint, pine, tea tree.

SCARS AND STRETCHMARKS
(promotes efficient healing of skin; essentially a preventative treatment)
Frankincense, lavender, neroli, patchouli. Also, infused oil of calendula.

SINUSITIS
Eucalyptus, lavender, peppermint, pine, tea tree.

SPOTS / PIMPLES
Lavender, tea tree.

SPRAINS AND BRUISES
Chamomile (preferably German), eucalyptus, lavender, marjoram (sweet), pine, rosemary, thyme (sweet).

SUNBURN
Chamomile (preferably German), lavender, rosemary, tea tree.

THROAT, SORE
Eucalyptus, frankincense, lavender, peppermint, sandalwood, tea tree.

TRAVEL/MOTION SICKNESS (See Nausea)

VARICOSE VEINS - to help reduce pain and inflammation
Cypress, frankincense, lavender.

Botanical and Common Names cross index

A

Anethum graveolens	Dill	61
Angelica archangelica	Angelica Seed	35
Apium graveolens	Celery Seed	49
Artemisia dracunculus	Tarragon	110

B

Betula alba	Birch White	41
Boswellia carterii	Frankincense	65

C

Calendula officinalis	Marigold (infusion)	83
Cananga odorata var. *genuina*	Ylang Ylang	115
Carum carvi	Caraway	45
Chamaemelum nobile	Chamomile, Roman	52
Cinnamomum camphora	Camphor - White	44
Cinnamomum camphora var. *galvescens*	Ho leaf	70
Cinnamomum zeylanicum	Cinnamon Leaf	53
Cistus ladaniferus	Ciste	54
Citrus aurantifolia	Lime	79
Citrus aurantium var. *amara*	Neroli	89
Citrus aurantium var. *amara*	Orange, Bitter	92
Citrus aurantium var. *amara,*also *C. aurantium* subsp. *aurantium*	Petitgrain	99
Citrus bergamia	Bergamot	40
Citrus limon	Lemon	77
Citrus reticulata	Mandarin	82
Citrus reticulata	Tangerine	109
Citrus sinensis	Orange, sweet	93
Citrus x *paradisi*	Grapefruit	69
Commiphora myrrha	Myrrh	87
Coriandrum sativum	Coriander	58
Cuminum cyminum	Cumin	59
Cupressus sempervirens	Cypress	60
Cymbopogon flexuosus	Lemongrass	78
Cymbopogon martinii	Palmarosa	95
Cymbopogon nardus	Citronella	55

D

Daucus carota	Carrot Seed	47

E

Elettaria cardomomum	Cardomom	46
Eucalyptus citriodora	Eucalyptus,Lemon-Scented	63
Eucalyptus globulus	Eucalyptus, Blue Gum	62

F

Ferula galbaniflua	Galbanum	66
Foeniculum vulgare	Fennel, Sweet	64

H

Hyssopus officinalis	Hyssop	71

I

Inula graveolens or *I. odorata*	Inula	72

J

Jasminum officinale	Jasmine Absolute	73
Juniperus communis	Juniper	74
Juniperus virginiana	Cedarwood, Virginian	48

L

Lavandula angustifolia	Lavender	76
Lavandula angustifolia x *L. latifolia*	Lavandin	75
Litsea cubeba	Litsea cubeba	81

M

Matricaria recutica	Chamomile, German	50
Melaleuca alternifolia	Tea Tree	111
Melaleuca leucadendron	Cajuput	43
Melaleuca viridiflora	Niaouli	90
Melissa officinalis	Melissa	86
Mentha piperita	Peppermint	98
Mentha spicata	Spearmint	107
Myristica fragrans	Nutmeg	91
Myrtus communis	Myrtle	88

O

Ocimum basilicum	Basil	37
Origanum majorana	Marjoram, sweet	85
Origanum vulgare	Origanum	94
Ormenis multicaulis	Chamomile, Maroc	51

P

Pelargonium graveolens	Geranium	67
Petroselinum sativum	Parsley Seed	96
Pimenta racemosa	Bay West Indian	38
Pimpinella anisum	Aniseed	36
Pinus sylvestris	Pine, Scots	100
Piper nigrum	Black Pepper	42
Pogostemon cablin	Patchouli	97

R

Rosa. damascena and several other varieties of *Rosa*	Rose Otto	103
Ravensara aromatica	Ravensara	101
Rosa centifolia and *R. damascena*	Rose Maroc Absolute	102
Rosmarinus officinalis	Rosemary	104

S

Salvia sclarea	Clary Sage	56
Santalum album	Sandalwood(AGMARK grade)	105
Satureja hortensis	Savory, Summer	106
Styrax tonkinensis	Benzoin Resinoid	39
Syzgium aromaticum	Clove	57

T

Tagetes minuta	Tagetes	108
Thymus mastichina	Marjoram, Spanish	84
Thymus vulgaris	Thyme, Sweet	112
Tilia cordata	Lime Blossom (Linden) Abs.	80

V

Valeriana fauriei	Valerian	113
Vetiveria zizanoides	Vetiver	114

Z

Zingiber officinale	Ginger	68

Essential Oils by Family Groups

Refer to chapter 5 Essential Oil Profiles for detailed information

A

Annonaceae	Ylang Ylang	115
Apiaceae (Umbelliferae)	Aniseed	36
	Caraway	45
	Carrot Seed	47
	Celery Seed	49
	Coriander	58
	Cumin	59
	Dill	61
	Galbanum	66
	Parsley Seed	96
	Angelica Seed	35
	Fennel, Sweet	64
Asteraceae	Chamomile, German	50
	Chamomile, Maroc	51
	Chamomile, Roman	52
	Inula	72
	Marigold (infusion)	83
	Tagetes	108
	Tarragon	110

B

Betulaceae	Birch White	41
Burseraceae	Frankincense	65
	Myrrh	87

C

Cistaceae	Ciste	54
Cupressaceae	Cedarwood, Virginian	48
	Cypress	60
	Juniper	74

G

Geraniaceae	Geranium	67
Gramineae	Palmarosa	95

L

Lamiaceae (Labiatae)	Basil	37
	Patchouli	97
	Savory, Summer	106
	Clary Sage	56
	Hyssop	71
	Lavandin	75
	Lavender	76
	Marjoram, Spanish	84
	Marjoram, sweet	85
	Melissa	86
	Origanum	94
	Peppermint	98
	Rosemary	104
	Spearmint	107
	Thyme, Sweet	112
Lauraceae	Camphor - White	44
	Cinnamon Leaf	53
	Ho leaf	70
	Litsea cubeba	81
	Ravensara	101

Select Bibliography

Essential Oils: Scientific Manuals

Watt, M. Plant Aromatics privately published, with updates 1999

Harris, B. Aromatherapy Database, published by Essential Oil Resource Consultants 1998

Botanical and Medicinal Information

Stodola, J and Volak, J. The Illustrated Book of Herbs, published by Octopus, 1984

Mabey, R. (Ed), The Complete New Herbal, published by Penguin, 1988.

Botanical Information

Johnson, A.T. and Smith H.A. Plant Names Simplified:
The Pronunciation, Derivation & Meaning
Published by Landsmans Bookshop Ltd., 1981.

Suggested General Reading

Wildwood, C.   Aromatherapy,   published by Bloomsbury, 1996
A black and white, condensed version of The Bloomsbury Encyclopaedia of
Aromatherapy, published by Bloomsbury, 1996 –   which is now out of print.
The full colour version of Aromatherapy is still available in the United States,
entitled "Encyclopedia of Aromatherapy"   by Healing Arts Press 1996

Wildwood, C.   Aroma Remedies,   published by Collins and Brown, 2000

Other Books by Chrissie Wildwood

Aromatherapy Made Easy   published by Thorsons, 1997
(Previously titled Holistic Aromatherapy published by Thorsons, 1992)

The Aromatherapy Massage Book   published by Thorsons, 1994

Flower Remedies for Women   published by Thorsons, 1994

The Book of Aromatherapy Blends   published by Thorsons, 1994
(Previously entitled Creative Aromatherapy published by Thorsons, 1993)

Flower Remedies – Natural Healing with Flower Essences
                          published by Element Books, 1992, 1998

Aromatherapy, Massage with Essential Oils
                          published by Element Books, 1991, 1997

Natural Healing – Practical Ways to Find Well-being and Inspiration
                          published by Piatkus, 2000
(Previously published in 1997 as "The Complete Guide to Reducing Stress")

Create Your Own Aromatherapy Perfumes Using Essential Oils
                          published by Piatkus, 1999
First published by Piatkus, 1995 as Create Your Own Perfumes Using Essential Oils

Useful Addresses

Suppliers of Quality Essential Oils

Amyris Essential Oils

PO Box 181
Harrogate.
North Yorkshire. HG2 0LX

Phone   01423   560 583
Fax   01423   522 603
Email   info@amyris.com
Web site www.amyris.com

Purple Flame

St. John's Spinney
New Arley
Warwickshire. CV7 8HA

Phone   01676   542 542
Fax   01676   540 777
Email   purple.flame@zetnet.co.uk
Web site www.purpleflame.co.uk

For Certificated organic essential oils (UK and Europe)

Florial France

Je International
42 Chemin Des Aubépines
06130 Grasse,
France.

Phone   0033   493 77 8819
Fax   0033   493 77 8878
Email   info@florial.com
Web site www.florial.com

The Essential Oils Trade Association

For advice and information on oils, trading ethics and legislation.
Works closely with Trading Standards and actively seeks to maintain standards.
Should you ever doubt the quality of an essential oil purchased in the UK, then this is
the organisation to contact.

EOTA

61 Clinton Lane
Kenilworth
Coventry. CV8 2BQ

Phone   01926   512 001
Fax   01926   512 001
Web site www.eota.org

Aromatherapy – Examining bodies

Contact the following organisations for lists of accredited aromatherapists and information about training courses

International Federation of Aromatherapists

IFA

182 Chiswick High Road	Telephone	0208	742 2605
London. W4 1TH	Fax	0208	742 2606
	Email		
	Web site www.int-fed-aromatherapy.co.uk		

The International Society for Professional Aromatherapists

ISPA

ISPA House	Telephone	01455	637 987
82 Ashby Road	Fax	01455	890 956
Hinkley	Email	lisabrown@ispa.demon.co.uk	
Leicestershire. LE10 1SN	Web site		

International Therapy Examination Council

ITEC

10-11 Heathfield Terrace	Telephone	0208	994 4141
Chiswick	Fax	0208	994 7880
London. W4 4JE	Email	info@itecworld.co.uk	
	Web site	www.itecworld.co.uk	

The Aromatherapy Organisation Council

AOC

PO Box 19834	Telephone	0208	251 7912
London. SE25 6WF	Fax	0208	251 7942
	Email		
	Web site www.aromatherapy-uk.org		

Massage Training

The Derby School of Holistic Massage

Contact: Mr M Bailey	Telephone	01332	299 133
32 Margaret Avenue	Fax		
Ilkeston	Email		
Derbyshire. DE7 5DD	Web site		

The Academy of on Site Massage

Avon Road	Telephone	01454	261 9000
Charfield	Fax	01454	261 9000
Wotton under Edge	Email all@onsitemassage.softnet.co.uk		
Gloucestershire. GL12 8TT	Web site www.aosm.co.uk		

Master Index

diarrhoea, 68, 89, 105
di-ethyl phthalate, 87
digestion, 110
digestive and respiratory ailments, 36
digestive complaints, 1
digestive problems, 58
digestive tonic, 101
digestive upsets, 95
Dill, 33, 61, 120, 122
disharmonious relationship, 25
disinfectant, 84, 90
distillation, 35, 36, 37, 38, 41, 42, 43,
    44, 45, 46, 48, 49, 50, 51, 52, 53,
    54, 55, 56, 58, 59, 60, 61, 62, 63,
    64, 66, 67, 68, 69, 70, 71, 72, 74,
    75, 76, 78, 83, 84, 85, 86, 87, 88,
    89, 90, 91, 94, 95, 96, 97, 98, 100,
    101, 103, 104, 105, 106, 107, 110,
    111, 112, 113, 114, 115
distilled, 38, 41, 44, 46, 57, 61, 69,
    77, 79, 87, 90, 91, 93, 102, 104,
    115
distilled water, 6, 15, 16, 17, 27, 38,
    46
diuretic, 27
Dominica, 38
douche, 18
downhearted, 13
Dr Jean Valnet, 1
Dr Jennes Kristott, 7
drowsiness, 56
dry inhalation, 13, 29, 61, 67
dry, flaky or irritated skin., 16

E

earache, 50, 52, 72, 76, 117
earthy, 25, 35, 47, 66, 95, 97, 113,
    114
East Indian, 78
eczema, 18, 41, 47, 50, 52, 76, 81,
    83, 97, 103
Egypt, 36, 44, 59
elderly people, 15, 101
elecampane, 72
emmenagogue, 87
emotion, 4, 15, 21, 28
emotional healing, 28, 29
emotional shock, 30
encapsulated essential oils, 1
Encens, 65
engendering, 60
enigmatic, 25

enlivening, 37, 46, 47, 53, 55, 67, 69,
    70, 78, 104
EOTA, 6, 125
epilepsy, 18, 64, 71, 104
ethyl glyco, 39
eucalyptus, 2, 6, 13, 18, 27, 28, 46,
    62, 63, 78, 85, 88, 98, 100, 101,
    104, 107, 111, 116, 117, 118, 119,
    120, 123
eugenol, 57
Europe, 35, 41, 45, 49, 50, 52, 58, 72,
    74, 80, 83, 94, 100, 106, 109, 110,
    113, 125
excessive menstruation, 60
exercise (moderate),1
expansive sensation, 60
expressed, 3, 6, 40, 77, 79, 93
eyes, 12, 18

F

face, 70
facial steam, 13
fainting, 98
fatal, 62
fatigue and nervous exhaustion, 117
fearfulness, 28, 31
feelings, 4
Fennel, 18, 25, 26, 47, 64, 120, 122
fever, 14, 40, 55, 70, 72, 78, 95, 98,
    103, 111, 117
fixed' or fatty oils, 2
flatulence, 35, 45, 46, 49, 59, 61, 64,
    66, 81, 85, 91, 98, 107
flies - to repel, 55
floral, 24, 25, 45, 56, 70, 73, 76, 80,
    89, 102, 116, 117
Florentine flask, 3
Florial France, 125
flu, 12, 37, 38, 39, 43, 45, 62, 68, 69,
    72, 79, 88
fluid retention, 27, 35, 41, 47, 49,
    61,64, 117, 118
food allergies, 18
fool's parsley, 33
foot / hand bath, 13
fortifying, 112
foxglove, 3
fractions, 44, 115
fragile capillaries, 83
fragrant grass, 25
France / French, 1, 18, 36, 47, 1,106,
    125

frankincense, 12, 17, 21, 22, 23, 24, 25, 27, 28, 30, 31, 35, 37, 39, 40, 41, 42, 46, 48, 51, 53, 54, 56, 57, 58, 60, 62, 65, 66, 68, 70, 72, 74, 76, 77, 81, 82, 87, 89, 92, 93, 99, 100, 102, 104, 105, 115, 116, 117, 118, 119, 120, 122

Friars Balsam, 39

fumigant, 14, 15, 38, 39, 43, 44, 53, 54, 57, 62, 63, 68, 71, 78, 81, 84, 88, 94, 106, 111, 112

fungal infections, 48

furocoumarin/s, 40

G

Galbanum, 59, 65, 66,110, 120, 122

gargles, 15

Gattefossé (Rene-Maurice), 1, 4

genus, 33

Geraniaceae, 67, 122

geraniol, 112

geranium, 5, 12, 16, 17, 22, 23, 24, 25, 27, 28, 37, 38, 40, 42, 45, 46, 47, 48, 50, 52, 55, 57, 58, 63, 64, 65, 66, 67, 69, 70, 71, 74, 76, 78, 79, 80, 81, 86, 87, 89, 90, 91, 93, 95, 97, 98, 99, 102, 104, 105, 115, 116, 117, 118, 121, 122

germs, 16

ginger, 2, 3, 22, 23, 24, 25, 27, 28, 31, 39, 40, 46, 68, 78, 87, 88, 93, 97, 116, 117, 118, 121, 123

gingivitis, 64, 87, 117

GLC analysis, 112

good nutrition, 1

gout, 35, 39, 47, 49, 100, 112

Gramineae, 55, 78, 95, 114, 122, 123

Grapefruit, 22, 23, 24, 27, 30, 40, 69, 71, 88, 120, 123

Grapeseed, 6, 11

grazes, 16, 63

Greece, 36

grief, 28, 29, 30

grounding, 24, 25, 35, 114

Guatemala, 78

gum disorders, 60, 64, 87

H

haemorrhoids, 60, 65, 74, 90, 117

hair tonic, 17, 38

hallucinations, 91

Harris, B, 124

hay fever, 62, 117

headache, 14, 21, 50, 51, 52, 55, 59, 62, 63, 76, 78, 85, 98, 102, 103, 104, 107, 112, 117

head-clearing, 43, 44, 46, 48, 62, 63, 65, 66, 84, 87, 88, 90, 98, 104, 111

headlice, 62, 67, 100, 104, 117

healthy hair, 104

heartburn, 117, 118

heartwood, 2, 105

heavy periods, 50

helichrysum, 28, 83, 101

hemlock, 33

herb, 37, 39, 45, 50, 52, 56, 58, 59, 61, 64, 66, 71, 72, 83, 84, 85, 86, 94, 96, 98, 106, 107, 108, 110, 112, 113

herbaceous, 24, 25, 35, 50, 51, 54, 56, 76, 94, 96, 97, 99, 106, 107, 112

herbal medicines, 2

hexane, 4

high blood pressure, 56, 77, 115

highly irritant, 37, 43, 53, 106

Ho leaf, 22, 23, 24, 44, 59, 70, 116, 120, 122

holistic, 1, 39, 50, 116

homoeopath, 18

hops, 118

hospitals, 90

hot compress, 14

hot flushes, 118

hunger, 4

hydrolat, 3

hydrosol, 3

Hyssop, 18, 71, 88, 120, 122

I

incense, 65

indecision, 28, 31

India, 36, 42, 46, 53, 73, 78, 87, 95, 97, 105, 114

indigestion, 35, 47, 49, 50, 53, 59, 61, 66, 68, 71, 78, 81, 82, 86, 87, 91, 93, 96, 98, 99, 117

Indonesia, 43, 57, 95, 114

infectious illness, 14, 38, 43, 44, 53, 54, 62, 63, 68, 71, 78, 81, 84, 88, 90, 94, 106, 111, 112

inflamed skin, 36, 39, 52, 66

inflammation, 14, 50, 60, 83, 117, 119

inhalation, 4, 13, 38, 44, 94, 106, 112
inhale, 43, 61, 64, 67
insect bites, 16, 18, 43, 50, 62, 76,
   83, 90, 111, 112, 118
insect repellent, 37, 44, 55, 57, 62,
   63, 75, 76, 78, 81, 97, 104, 108,
   118
insomnia, 21, 50, 51, 52, 76, 80, 82,
   85, 86, 99, 102, 103, 105, 113,
   114, 115, 118
instincts, 4
International Federation of
   Aromatherapists, 126
International Therapy Examination
   Council, 126
intestinal parasites, 106
intoxicating, 24, 25, 73, 80, 115
intuition, 4
Inula, 72, 120, 122
invigorating, 24, 25, 41, 74, 90, 107
irregular menstruation, 56, 86, 103
irritability, 18, 28
irritable bowel syndrome, 98
irritant / irritate / irritation, 5, 38, 45,
   48, 53, 55, 57, 62, 63, 64, 67, 68,
   69, 74, 76, 77, 78, 79, 84, 86, 90,
   91, 93, 96, 98, 102, 104, 106,
   107,109
Italy, 40
itching, 19
itchy skin, 83

J

jangled nervous, 99
Japan, 1, 41, 44, 74
jasmine, 4, 18, 22, 23, 24, 25, 28, 31,
   39, 42, 45, 46, 48, 52, 54, 56, 58,
   70, 73, 89, 92, 102, 105, 114, 115,
   116, 117, 118, 120, 123
Jojoba, 11, 15, 102
juniper, 17, 22, 23, 24, 25, 27, 28, 30,
   31, 39, 40, 43, 48, 54, 56, 58, 60,
   65, 69, 74, 76, 77, 85, 87, 100,
   111, 116, 117, 118, 120, 122

K

Karl von Linné, 33
ketones, 108
kidney disease, 74
Korea, 74

L

labdanum, 54
Lamiaceae (Labiatae),37, 56, 71, 75,
   76, 84, 85, 86, 94, 97, 98, 104,
   106, 107, 112, 122
laryngitis, 39, 65, 73, 76, 87, 105, 112
Lauraceae, 44, 53, 70, 81, 101, 122
lavandin, 38, 43, 51, 54, 59, 75, 84,
   88, 90, 91, 92, 93, 95, 106, 107,
   112, 120, 122
Lavandula angustifolia, 5, 75, 76, 120
lavender, 2, 4, 5, 12, 13, 14, 16, 17,
   18, 21, 22, 23, 24, 25, 27, 28, 30,
   31, 38, 40, 42, 43, 46, 47, 49, 50,
   51, 52, 54, 56, 57, 59, 60, 62, 64,
   65, 66, 69, 70, 71, 72, 74, 75, 76,
   77, 78, 79, 82, 83, 84, 85, 86, 87,
   88, 89, 90, 91, 92, 93, 94, 95, 97,
   98, 99, 100, 101, 102, 104, 105,
   106, 107, 108, 110, 111, 112, 113,
   114, 116, 117, 118, 119, 120, 122
lemon, 2, 6, 17, 22, 23, 24, 25, 27,
   28, 30, 31, 35, 36, 37, 39, 40, 43,
   44, 45, 48, 51, 54, 62, 63,71, 75,
   77, 78, 84, 86, 88, 90, 98, 106,
   108, 110, 111, 116, 117, 120, 123
lemongrass, 22, 23, 24, 25, 26, 27,
   28, 30, 31, 37, 40, 55, 61, 75, 78,
   81, 82, 86, 87, 95, 104, 112, 114,
   117, 118, 120, 123
lethargy, 42
libido, 4, 28, 31, 118
light-headedness, 114
limbic system, 4
Lime, Lime Blossom, Linden, 3, 22,
   23, 24, 27, 28, 30, 31, 37, 69, 75,
   79, 80, 115, 117, 120, 121, 123
linalol, 112
Linnaeus, 33
Litsea cubeba, 81, 121, 122
liver congestion, 47, 49
loss of appetite, 42, 68, 95
loss of periods, 48, 49, 59, 61, 64, 66,
   74
lotions, 15, 41
lymphatic drainage, 69, 117

M

Mabey, R, 124
maceration, 83
Madagascar, 42, 44, 95, 101, 115
Malaysia, 42, 43, 97

132

mandarin, 17, 22, 23, 24, 25, 27, 28, 30, 31, 65, 78, 80, 81, 82, 86, 97, 102, 109, 113, 118, 120, 123
Marigold, 83, 108, 120, 122
marjoram, 22, 24, 27, 28, 50, 60, 61, 62, 84, 85, 90, 98, 100, 111, 112, 116, 117, 118, 119, 121, 122
masculine, 97, 105
massage, 1, 2, 6, 7, 9, 10, 11, 13, 15, 17, 21, 26, 27, 28, 29, 36, 39, 41, 53, 54, 56, 65, 69, 72, 92, 99, 103, 108, 111, 112, 117, 115
massage oil, 27, 42, 47, 48, 56, 59, 62, 65, 66, 67, 70, 74, 76, 78, 82, 85, 86, 87, 93, 97, 100, 101, 105
massage oil blend, 42, 47, 48, 56, 59, 65, 66, 70, 74, 76, 78, 82, 85, 86, 87, 93, 97, 100, 105
Massage Training, 126
mature skin, 47, 65, 66, 70
Maury, Marguerite, 1
measles, 62, 63
medical herbalist, 3, 18, 50
meditation, 54, 60, 65, 66
Mediterranean, 54, 56, 59, 60, 61, 71, 76, 77, 82, 84, 85, 86, 88, 89, 92, 93, 96, 98, 99, 104, 107, 109, 112
melaleuca, 43
Melissa (Lemon Balm) , 5, 26, 28, 30, 33, 86, 112, 116, 117, 119, 121, 122
memory, 4
menopausal distress, 56, 60, 67
menopausal symptoms, 118
menstrual cramp, 14
menstrual pain, 52
menstrual problems, 118
menstruation, 35, 65, 71, 74, 76, 84, 85, 87, 103, 104, 108
mental alertness, 22
mental fatigue, 13, 37, 42, 46, 58, 68, 98, 104, 118
mental stimulant, 24, 25, 27
mexican, 83, 108
Mexico, 36
Middle East, 37, 39, 54, 66, 73, 87
middle notes, 22, 38
migraine, 35, 50, 55, 56, 59, 76, 85, 86, 98, 107, 118
mild depression, 37, 40, 54, 56, 67, 69, 70, 73, 76, 77, 79, 89, 92, 93, 97, 101, 102, 103, 105, 112, 114, 115
milk flow, 49

milk production., 18
mimosa, 48, 56, 76, 114
minor burns, 18
minty, 25
Molucca Islands, 91
mood, 24, 25
mood enhancement, 13, 15
Mood Swings, 28, 30
mood-elevating, 36, 40, 73, 93
mood-enhancing, 21, 51, 80
mother's milk, 61
mouth, 46, 64, 87, 98
mouth ulcers, 15, 118
mouthwash, 15, 46, 64, 107
mucous membranes, 38, 53, 57, 94, , 106112
muscular aches and pains, 1,12, 14, 21, 36, 37, 38, 41, 42, 43, 44, 50, 56, 58, 62, 63, 66, 68, 73, 74, 75, 76, 78, 84, 85, 90, 91, 94, 98, 100, 101, 104, 107, 112, 114, 118
musky, 24, 25, 54, 58, 59, 73, 97, 105, 113
Myristicaceae, 91, 123
myrrh, 39, 62, 77, 78, 87, 93, 97, 105, 116, 117, 118, 120, 122
Myrtaceae, 38, 43, 57, 62, 63, 88, 90, 111, 123
Myrtle, 22, 23, 24, 28, 30, 31, 71, 88, 101, 116, 117, 118, 121, 123
Mysore, 105

N

nappy rash, 83
narcissus, 4
nasal congestion, 13
nature identical, 5
nausea, 42, 68, 76, 86, 91, 98, 102, 105, 107, 118, 119
nebulizer, 14
neck, 6, 12, 29, 70
Neroli, 6, 12, 17, 21, 22, 23, 24, 25, 28, 30, 31, 33, 37, 39, 40, 46, 48, 50, 52, 54, 56, 58, 65, 67, 68, 69, 70, 74, 76, 77, 79, 82, 86, 89, 91, 92, 93, 96, 97, 99, 102, 114, 116, 117, 118, 119, 120, 123
nervous exhaustion / fatigue, 35, 45, 46, 49, 53, 54, 58, 59, 68, 69, 71, 78, 79, 84, 86, 91, 95, 96, 97, 99, 100, 101, 104, 112, 114
nervous indigestion, 13, 35, 45, 110, 113

saffrol, 44
sage, 18, 24, 28, 56, 77
sandalwood, 2, 5, 12, 17, 22, 23, 25, 27, 28, 30, 39, 40, 41, 42, 48, 54, 58, 60, 61, 64, 65, 67, 68, 70, 72, 73, 74, 77, 80, 82, 87, 92, 95, 97, 102, 103, 105, 113, 114, 115, 116, 117, 118, 119, 121, 123
Santalaceae, 105, 123
Savory, Summer, 106, 121, 122
scabies, 45, 76, 78, 98, 100, 104, 112
scalds, 116
scalp, 38, 97
scars, 65, 66, 119
sciatica, 49, 96
Scots pine, 22, 23, 54, 69
sea salt, 112
sebum, 17
sedative, 21, 27, 56
seeds, 11, 35, 36, 45, 46, 47, 49, 58, 59, 64, 96, 101
seizure, 18, 64, 71, 104
sensitise, 39, 53, 63, 93, 100, 115
sensitive skin, 3, 9, 10, 11, 12, 15, 18, 19, 48, 51, 53, 55, 64, 67, 68, 73, 78, 81, 86, 91, 92, 93, 100, 102, 104, 107
sensuous, 82, 103, 115
sexual desire, 44, 85
shampoos, 41
shelf-life, 69, 77, 79, 82, 109
shock, 28, 30
Siberia, 35, 80
Sicily, 40
sinusitis, 43, 72, 98, 100, 101, 107, 112, 119
skin - tonics, 16
skin absorption, 4, 9
skin and hair care, 16, 41, 47, 50, 52, 54, 55, 60, 65, 66, 67, 74, 76, 77, 89, 95, 97, 99, 102, 103, 104, 105, 114
skin applications, 17, 35, 37, 40, 42, 52, 53, 56, 64, 65, 73, 74, 77, 80, 81, 85, 92, 93, 98, 104, 106, 112
skin cancer, 92
skin complaints, 13
Skin Cream, 13, 16, 50
skin eruptions, 14, 21
skin infections, 62
skin irritation, 6, 43, 52, 93
skin perfume, 15, 102
skin problems, 1, 12
skin rashes, 50

skin sensitiser, 72
skin tonics, 16, 17
skin type, 16
skin ulcers, 54, 66
skin-care treatments, 9, 11, 16
sleep, 1, 4
sleeplessness, 18
sluggish circulation, 27
solar plexus, 29
soles of the feet, 29
solvent, 39, 54, 73, 80, 83, 87, 89, 102, 108
Somali, 87
soothe the mind, 21
soothing, 24, 25, 39, 42, 50, 51, 72, 80, 82, 89, 102, 103, 105
sore and cracked nipples, 83
sore throat, 15, 43, 68, 71, 77, 87, 90, 100, 105, 112
sores, 66, 97
South America, 70, 97, 108
Spain, 36, 62
spasmodic cough, 98
spearmint, 22, 23, 25, 26, 27, 29, 30, 31, 107, 116, 117, 118, 121, 122
species, 33, 70, 85, 87, 105
specific name, 33
spices, 25, 38, 42, 47, 49, 57, 58, 61, 68, 92, 102, 103, 115
spicy, 24, 35, 36, 37, 38, 42, 45, 46, 47, 53, 57, 58, 59, 61, 68, 71, 91, 96, 101, 106
spikenard, 28, 30
spots, 119
sprains, 14, 44, 50, 62, 85, 98, 116, 119
Sri Lanka, 53, 55, 114
St John's wort, 41
stabilising effect, 71
standardised oils, 5
steam distillation, 3, 4, 47, 65, 74, 79, 81, 99, 108
steam Inhalation, 9, 13,18, 26, 39, 43, 53, 72, 107
steam treatments, 13
stiff joints, 43
stimulates menstruation, 45, 47, 55, 66
stimulating, 24, 25, 36, 38, 42, 43, 45, 54, 57, 58, 59, 61, 64, 68, 94, 95, 106, 110, 112
stings, 16, 43, 50, 62, 66, 76, 90, 111, 112
Stodola, J, 124

vaporisation, 14
vaporising blend, 27, 35, 36, 37, 39, 40, 44, 45, 53, 55, 57, 60, 62, 63, 69, 71, 73, 75, 77, 79, 80, 81, 84, 90, 91, 92, 94, 96, 98, 106, 108, 110, 113
varicose veins, 60, 83, 90, 119
vegetable oil, 7, 9, 13, 39
veruccae, 111
vetiver, 2, 22, 23,25, 26, 28, 35, 40, 48, 54, 56, 65, 67, 68, 74, 76, 92, 95, 97, 99, 105, 113, 114, 115, 116, 121, 123
vitality, 1, 9
vitamin E, 6, 7, 11
Volak, J, 124
volatile solvents, 7

W

warming, 24, 27, 35, 36, 38, 39, 42, 45, 46, 47, 50, 52, 53, 54, 57, 58, 59, 61, 64, 65, 68, 71, 73, 74, 85, 87, 91, 93, 94, 96, 97, 101, 102, 103, 104, 106, 110, 112, 114, 115

Watt, M, 124
weeping eczema, 74
well-being, 103
West Indian, 78
West Indian bay, 38

West Indian sandalwood, 105
West Indies, 38, 68, 91
wheatgerm, 7
White birch, 41
white, brown and yellow camphor, 44
whooping cough, 71, 72
wild plants, 112
Wild Thyme, 112
winter blues, 67
witchazel, 16
wormwood, 33
worry, 28, 30
wounds, 27, 50, 52, 54, 60, 62, 65, 66, 71, 74, 87, 90, 95, 97, 100, 111, 112

Y

Yemen, 87
Ylang Ylang,17, 22, 23, 25, 27, 28, 30, 31, 38, 39, 42, 46, 47, 48, 50, 53, 57, 67, 68, 72, 77, 79, 80, 82, 89, 91, 92, 102, 105, 114, 115, 116, 117, 118, 119, 120, 122

Z

zest, 77
Zingiberaceae, 46, 68, 123